It's the Calories, Not the Carbs

IT'S STILL THE CALORIES, NOT THE CARBS...

When "It's the Calories, Not the Carbs" was first written, the goal was to educate confused consumers about the dangers of fad dieting, the naturalness of intuitive eating, and that all foods can fit into a healthful diet. Eating well and living well was the book's mantra, with most of the information provided based on the scientifically supported advice presented in the 2000 *Dietary Guidelines* and corresponding Food Guide Pyramid.

Since that time, a new set of *Dietary Guidelines* has been introduced — but that doesn't mean you have to toss your copy of "It's the Calories, Not the Carbs." The truth is, the new *Guidelines* incorporate many of the sentiments captured in the previous version and outlined in the book. The overwhelming conclusion remains: It's still the calories, not the carbs, that count. And you don't even have to actually count the calories to make it work! Furthermore, complex carbohydrates, particularly whole grains, have risen to a whole new level of importance in the *Guidelines*.

This new introduction aims to provide an overview of the new *Guidelines*, including how they stack up to the previous *Guidelines* and the recommendations provided in the book. In the end, whether your personal health goal is to become an intuitive eater, achieve and/or maintain your natural healthy weight, become more active, have more energy, or just improve your overall health and fitness,

"It's the Calories, Not the Carbs" remains a valuable resource and tool to help you make lasting, healthful lifestyle changes and achieve your overall goals.

THE HISTORY BEHIND THE 2005 *DIETARY GUIDELINES*

In January 2005, the government released the newest version of the *Dietary Guidelines*. This report, officially called the *Dietary Guidelines for Americans 2005*, is revamped every five years through the joint efforts of the Department of Health and Human Services (HHS) and the Department of Agriculture (USDA). Experts review the most current scientific and medical research, which results in nutritional and dietary information and guidelines for the general public ages 2 years and older. The intent of this report is to provide science-based advice to promote health and to reduce risk for major chronic diseases through diet and physical activity.

Basically, this means the *Dietary Guidelines* were designed to help Americans make informed choices about food and physical activity, so they can live healthier lives. It is used to update the USDA's Food Guidance System — what was once known as the Food Guide Pyramid and has been most recently reintroduced as MyPyramid.

THE 2000 VS. 2005 *DIETARY GUIDELINES*

There have been a number of changes in the 2005 *Dietary Guidelines* from previous years. However, the *Guidelines* continue to focus on the importance of grain foods in our diet. We need three daily servings of whole grains, such as whole wheat pasta, whole wheat bread, or whole grain cereal, with the rest of the recommended grains coming from enriched or whole grain products.

The *Guidelines* also are more specific regarding exercise

recommendations, suggesting that 60 minutes of moderate to vigorous exercise are needed most days to avoid gaining weight as we age, and that those who were once overweight may need to exercise more — for 60 to 90 minutes a day — if they don't want the pounds to slip back on. While incorporating exercise is key in any daily routine, we are not in full agreement with these recommendations and will address this issue later in this introduction.

More specifically, the 2005 *Dietary Guidelines* recommend that we:

- Consume a variety of foods within and among the basic food groups while staying within energy needs.

- Control calorie intake to manage body weight.

- Be physically active every day.

- Increase daily intake of fruits and vegetables, whole grains, and nonfat or low-fat milk and milk products.

- Choose fats wisely for good health.

- Choose carbohydrates wisely for good health.

- Choose and prepare foods with little salt.

- If you drink alcoholic beverages, do so in moderation.

- Keep food safe to eat.

The *Guidelines* discourage consumption of too much sugar, and plant and fish oils are given new emphasis for the positive effects they have on heart health. The *Guidelines* can be viewed online at *www.healthierus.gov/dietaryguidelines*.

2000:	2005:
WEIGHT Aim for a healthy weight.	WEIGHT Maintain weight in a healthy range by balancing calories from food and beverages with calories expended.
EXERCISE Be physically active each day.	EXERCISE To help manage body weight, engage in 60 minutes of moderate to vigorous activity on most days. To sustain weight loss, increase to up to 90 minutes.
FOOD GROUPS Let the Food Guide Pyramid inform your choices.	FOOD GROUPS Choose a variety of nutrient-dense foods within and among the basic food groups.
FRUITS, VEGETABLES, GRAINS, SUGAR Choose a variety of fruits and vegetables and grains daily, especially whole grains. Moderate intake of sugars.	FRUITS, VEGETABLES, GRAINS, SUGAR Choose fiber-rich fruits, vegetables, and whole grains. Consume three or more ounces of whole grain products per day. Consume two cups of fruit and two and a half cups of vegetables per day.
FAT Choose a diet that is low in saturated fat and cholesterol and moderate in total fat.	FAT Total fat intake should be from 20 percent to 35 percent of calories with most fats coming from sources such as fish, nuts, and vegetable oils. Consume less than 10 percent of calories from saturated fats and keep trans fats as low as possible.
SODIUM Choose and prepare foods with less salt.	SODIUM Consume less than 2,300 milligrams or about 1 teaspoon daily. In general, greater consumption of nutrient-dense foods – foods packed with vitamins, minerals, fiber, and other nutrients but lower in calories – is encouraged.

We are pleased to see the *Dietary Guidelines* emphasize that, when it comes to weight control, it is calories that count — not the proportions of fat, carbohydrates, and protein in the diet. But in some ways, the focus is problematic, especially considering the new Pyramid scheme, discussed below. While the new *Guidelines* and Pyramids are more individualized, they dramatically increase focus on calories alone, especially considering the comment at the bottom of each of the 12 Pyramids: "This calorie level is only an estimate of your needs. Monitor your body weight to see if you need to adjust your calorie intake." The implication is that the only way we can tell if we are getting the right amount of calories is if we have a scale. It misses entirely a person's ability to regulate their weight internally.

Fortunately, the *Guidelines* recognize that it is not the carbs that make a person fat, but eating more than the body needs, of any food, that has the potential to add weight to the body. This is important given the recent low-carb craze. The government confirms that carbohydrates have an important place in a healthy diet and in maintaining a healthy weight.

The recommendations for the percentages of fats (20 percent to 35 percent) and carbohydrates (45 percent to 65 percent) in the diet offer considerable flexibility and room for differences in individual needs. The upper range of the recommendation for protein (10 percent to 35 percent) is probably way too high. For instance, the recommendation for an 18-year-old, sedentary woman is 1,800 calories per day. If she took in 35 percent of her calories in protein, she would be consuming 157 grams of protein per day. Her actual needs would be closer to 44 grams protein per day. When you consider the diets of the most long-lived populations are fairly low in protein, we recommend aiming for the lower end of the protein range and the middle-to-upper end of the carbohydrate range. Additionally, the leanest populations in the world consume high-carbohydrate, low-fat diets. So if weight is a concern for you, consider consuming a diet that is in the upper end of the carbohydrate recommendations (and practice intuitive eating).

We also agree with the recommendations for reducing trans fat consumption.

MyPyramid

The Food Guide Pyramid was given an overhaul as a result of the new *Guidelines* as well and was unveiled April 2005. The USDA replaced the old version with a vertically striped edition that gives specific advice about how much and what kinds of foods the average person should eat each day (see Table 2). In fact, it provides 12 different versions depending on your calorie needs. Individuals log on to the new USDA Web site, *www.mypyramid.com,* enter their age, sex, and physical activity, and get a somewhat personalized "food pyramid."

Unfortunately, the new Pyramid no longer stands alone since there are no icons or text listing what the different vertical sections mean. The new Pyramid has six vertical stripes, each one representing various food groups and getting progressively wider at the base. Reading across, the comparative width of the stripes represents the balance of food groups. Reading up and down, the narrow point of the Pyramid and the wide base represent different total calorie requirements based on age, sex, and activity level.

When we say it's the calories, not the carbs, that count, we mean while it's ultimately the calories, in theory, that affect weight gain/ loss/maintenance, there is no need to actually count calories. The new MyPyramid scheme is entirely too focused on calories. Truth be told, there is so much variation in individual metabolic needs (and basal metabolism), as well as wide variation in calorie expenditure individuals may have in performing 30, 60, or 60+ minutes per day in activity, that the calorie estimates are not much better than guessing. Plus, the formula does not include weight. Weight plays a huge role in determining calorie expenditure at rest and during activity, and thus should be incorporated into any eating recommendations.

However, once again, we know people can regulate their weight through intuitive eating, which is discussed below and in chapter five. This goes unnoticed in the new Pyramid, as it did in the previous one.

In addition, the wide variation in macronutrient composition (20 percent to 35 percent fat, 45 percent to 65 percent carbs, 10 percent to 35 percent protein) of the 2005 *Dietary Guidelines* does not really conform with the new Pyramid schemes. For each of the 12 different Pyramids, the serving recommendations are predominantly grains, fruits, and veggies — all low fat. The milk/dairy and meat recommendations also are "low" fat, "non" fat, or "lean." These food groups represent the major sources of calories. Even if the discretionary calories were heavy on the fat, it would be nearly impossible to approach 35 percent of total calories from fat (unless the person is very physically active and has a very high calorie intake, which pertains to a very small percentage of the population). Most fairly sedentary people, or even moderately active, will only have a discretionary calorie allowance of about 8 percent to 15 percent of total calories. It is almost impossible to see how anyone could consume 35 percent of total calories from fat (or protein) if they actually followed the Pyramid recommendations, even if almost all discretionary calories came from fat (or protein).

On the positive side, the new Pyramid uses "cups" as a measurement instead of "servings," which most people didn't understand. This allows people to better conceptualize average serving sizes. It also includes a figure walking up steps to remind us that exercise is an important component to health and nutrition.

The USDA Web site includes an interactive tool that allows consumers to assess their current state of nutrition and exercise. Unfortunately, perhaps those who need the information the most, those with lower incomes and the elderly, may not have access to a computer.

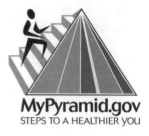

MyPyramid.gov
STEPS TO A HEALTHIER YOU

WHOLE GRAINS VS. REFINED GRAINS

The *2005 Dietary Guidelines* recommend Americans "consume three or more ounce equivalents of whole grain products per day, with the rest of the recommended grain servings coming from enriched or whole grain products." In general, at least half the grains should come from whole grains.

We are all for whole grains and highlight their specific health benefits in chapter two. Research shows whole grain foods are associated with lower rates of heart disease, diabetes, and certain cancers, and may help with better weight control. Despite these well-documented health benefits, Americans average less than one serving of whole grains per day! Therefore, we strongly support the new *Dietary Guidelines* recommendation for more whole grain consumption. And we also support the consumption of enriched grain products, as they can be good sources of folic acid, B vitamins, iron, and antioxidants.

However, to achieve the more ambitious goal of at least three servings of whole grain products per day, the *Dietary Guidelines* recommend substituting whole grains for refined grains. This gives the impression there is no place in the diet for refined grains. While it may make sense for some to choose more whole grain alternatives, particularly in an effort to increase consumption of dietary fiber, remember refined grain products also have significant health benefits. Many people are losing out on these health benefits due to the "bad carb" label that has been slapped on these foods as a result of the low-carb diet craze.

The blame refined grains have received for a number of health problems, such as diabetes and excessive weight gain, is not uniformly justified by published research. Many large-scale studies show no link between refined grain intake and either relative body weight or incidence of diabetes. And contrary to prevailing dogma, relative body weights and obesity prevalence, for example, tend to be lowest in people consuming high-carbohydrate diets, even high in refined grains. The most likely explanation is that people who consume lots of carbohydrates tend to consume more fiber-rich foods as well (i.e., high-carbohydrate diets tend to be higher in both whole and refined grain foods). The higher fiber intake may be the key factor in terms of these lower weights.

In sum, consuming more whole grain products is definitely a good idea. But avoiding refined grain products because they are "poor" nutrition choices is not justified. All foods can fit in a balanced diet, including all kinds of grain products.

EATING HEALTHY: PUTTING THE *GUIDELINES* INTO PRACTICE

Mark Twain once said, "The only way to keep your health is to eat what you don't want, drink what you don't like, and do what you'd rather not." Those who feel discouraged by the seemingly daunting task of implementing the new *Guidelines* just might agree with him!

However, healthy eating is actually not nearly as difficult as Mark Twain once said. You may find healthy eating can even be fun. But it does not have to be perfect. Remember, healthy eating is a dynamic process. Some days you may eat nine servings of fruits and vegetables, other days you may get four. Some days you will get in three servings of whole grains and three of refined grains, other days you might find you are getting all of one or the other. Don't worry. The important thing is to use the *Dietary Guidelines* as just that — guidelines, not rules for eating that feel like yet another diet.

This means you need to think in terms of "how can I get in another fruit or vegetable today." Not, "It's 4 p.m. and I've only eaten one fruit, there is no way I can eat eight more so I might as well forget it." Progress, not perfection, needs to be the goal. And remember, increasing your intake of fruits and vegetables from three servings a day (what most Americans get) to five servings a day will provide more benefits than going from seven servings a day to nine. So, small changes add up to big benefits!

WHAT A MENU FOLLOWING THE **2005** *GUIDELINES* LOOKS LIKE

What would it look like if you ate according to the new *Guidelines*? Following is a menu for one day that meets the requirements for a person consuming 2,000 calories. Make sure to note most relatively active women and men need to consume more than 2,000 calories a day.

2,000-CALORIE MENU
  BREAKFAST
    1 cup whole grain cereal
    1 cup low-fat milk
    1/2 cup strawberries

LUNCH

1 turkey sandwich

    2 slices regular whole wheat bread

    2 ounces lean turkey breast lunchmeat

    2 lettuce leaves

    1 tomato slice

    1 teaspoon mayonnaise

10 baby carrots

1 cup low-fat yogurt

SNACK

1 medium orange

DINNER

3 ounces baked fish cooked in 1 teaspoon olive oil

1/2 sweet potato with 1 teaspoon butter

1 cup cooked carrots

2 dinner rolls

1 green salad with 1 tablespoon low-fat dressing

SNACK

1 cup grapes

8 ounces fat-free milk

Plus approximately 270"discretionary calories" such as:

1 6-ounce glass of wine

1 cookie

DISCRETIONARY CALORIE ALLOWANCE

According to the 2005 *Dietary Guidelines*, we are allowed to have "discretionary calories." These are calories that are available "only when the amount of calories used to meet recommended nutrient intake is less than the total daily calorie expenditure."

They are provided to allow for foods such as butter, salad dressing, a cookie or two, or maybe a glass of wine. The caveat is these discretionary calories are allowed only when a person's full calorie allotment has not been used up by choosing foods from the other groups that are higher in calories. In other words, to get the discretionary calories, people must eat nutrient-dense foods that let them meet their recommended nutrient intake without using their full calorie allotment.

Discretionary calories break down to:

- 132 calories if you are consuming 1,600 calories per day
- 267 calories if you are consuming 2,000 calories per day
- 648 calories if you are consuming 3,200 calories per day

This means if you need 2,000 calories per day, and you have consumed all of the recommended foods, you can enjoy a 6-ounce glass of wine and a cookie. This may sound suspiciously like a diet to you, but it is important to be able to use eating guidelines without falling back into a diet mentality.

The whole concept of discretionary calories means that all foods fit! So often, people believe they cannot be healthy if they eat a piece of cake or a candy bar. With discretionary calories, you can choose nutrient-dense foods, or not, and still be contributing to your health.

The idea of discretionary calories is a positive one in that it gives people some flexibility with food; however, as presented earlier, this again places too much emphasis on calorie counting. Because the discretionary calories vary so much among the different Pyramids (in terms of calorie totals), and considering some foods have both nondiscretionary and discretionary calories in them, these discretionary calories become very confusing and tedious to keep track of. Instead, consumers should consider the intuitive eating approach, which is discussed below and in chapter five of this book.

While the *Guidelines* recognize calories count, the *Guidelines* also are geared to help you eat healthy without having to calorie count. In other words, the *Guidelines* and your body figure out the calories so you don't have to. The recommendations provided in "It's the Calories, Not the Carbs" still hold true in terms of showing you how to eat healthfully without counting calories.

Knowing How Much You Need to Eat

Research shows "human beings are born with the innate ability to regulate their food intake and healthy bodies come in all shapes and sizes." (ref – JR) Healthy babies are able to naturally self-regulate food intake by eating when hungry and stopping when full, resulting in adequate nutrition to support their growth and health. (Crawford and Shapiro, 1991; Johnson and Birch, 1994; Rose and Mayer, 1968). And so are adults!

The beauty of the 2005 *Guidelines*, as well as the 2000 version, is they both are structured in such a way to allow for flexibility in terms of how you use them. One of the most successful ways to embrace the *Guidelines,* follow your calorie needs, and take the stress out of eating is the concept of intuitive (or attuned) eating. With intuitive eating, you will find a natural, gentler way of eating healthy which suggests you do not need to exert a great deal of control over what and how much we eat. In fact, too much control can be counterproductive:

> "This way of looking at food, coldly, with distance and distrust becomes self-perpetuating. Our current situation is not going to lead to furthering the enjoyment and experience of food. And that's a real problem, because the experience and enjoyment of food brings you more self-awareness, and self-awareness will

bring self-control." (M. Stacy, 1994)

Self-control can arise naturally when we truly enjoy and experience food. According to many experts, the first place to start is by paying attention to your body's signals of hunger and satiety. In other words, use your body to tell you when to eat and when to quit eating.

Remember, satisfaction results, in part, from *knowing* size when you are hungry and eating in response to that hunger. This makes sense. The primary purpose of hunger is to signal the body needs to eat. The goal of eating is to relieve hunger. If you are not in touch with hunger, or aware of how hungry you are, how will you know how much to eat and/or when to stop eating?

"It's the Calories, Not the Carbs" can help you begin to understand how to eat when hungry and quit when satisfied. Combine this with an eating plan that will help you get the nutrients your body needs, and you are well on your way to a healthy lifestyle.

PHYSICAL ACTIVITY RECOMMENDATIONS IN THE 2005 *GUIDELINES*

The key recommendations of the new *Dietary Guidelines* are very much in line with the recommendations we make in chapter six (The Importance of Physical Activity and Fitness in Health). Specifically, the *Guidelines* recommend:

- Engage in regular physical activity and reduce sedentary activities to promote health, psychological well-being, and a healthy body weight.
- Achieve physical fitness by including cardiovascular conditioning, stretching exercises for flexibility, and resistance exercises or calisthenics for muscle strength and endurance.

In keeping with these key recommendations, we describe in chapter six important differences between physical activity and fitness and provide suggestions for becoming more physically active. We also include easy-to-perform fitness assessment tools so you can track changes in cardiovascular and muscular fitness and flexibility.

The unique aspect of the new *Guidelines* is the specific recommendations for how much physical activity is needed to achieve **three** different goals. Below we have stated each of the three new specific recommendations, with our take on the recommendation after each.

1. To reduce risk of chronic disease in adulthood: *Engage in at least 30 minutes* of moderate-intensity physical activity, above usual activity, at work or in home on most days of the week.

    OUR TAKE: As a baseline, this recommendation is generally fine and is similar to the Surgeon General's recommendation released in 1996, which has been the prevailing public health message for physical activity since that time. The key difference is the "above usual activity" qualification, which did not appear in the original Surgeon General's recommendation. This might cause some confusion for many adults because "usual activity" is somewhat nebulous. In chapter six, we use the recommendation of the National Academy of Science's Institute of Medicine, released in 2002, which encourages adults to aim for a goal of 60 minutes per day of at least moderate-intensity activity. This more ambitious goal was designed to promote both health and cardiovascular fitness benefits and is why we decided to use it. Since most people will have at least some moderate-intensity activity in their "usual activity," adding 30 minutes to this baseline will actually move people closer to this 60-minutes-per-day recommendation. It is important to note that the

60-minutes-per-day recommendation pertains to all moderate-intensity activity, including usual daily activities. When you consider that moderate-intensity activity elevates your resting pulse by no more than about 20 to 40 beats per minute and includes such activities as brisk walking, gardening, a number of household chores, and recreational activities such as dancing and golf, getting between 30 and 60 minutes per day of moderate-intensity activity on most days of the week is probably doable for most adults.

2. To help manage body weight and prevent gradual, unhealthy weight gain in adulthood: Engage in approximately *60 minutes* of moderate-to-vigorous-intensity activity on most days of the week while not exceeding caloric intake requirements.

OUR TAKE: We encourage physical activity and provide information in chapter six on moving toward incorporating more vigorous physical activity into your life. It should be emphasized vigorous activity does not mean exhaustive! In fact, vigorous activity includes such activities as aerobic dance, bicycling, jogging, swimming, and playing racquet sports. To qualify as vigorous, your heart rate has to be elevated by only about 40 beats per minute above your resting baseline; that is well below maximum. The problem we have with this recommendation is it is focused on body weight control. First, the statement implies physical activity is merely a means to an end. Second, the statement implicitly encourages calorie counting. We advocate (chapter five, How Much Do I Need to Eat?) a non-restrictive, non-calorie-counting approach to eating. We also encourage physical activity for its own intrinsic value and not solely for its calorie-burning potential (there are no exercise "calorie equivalents" charts in our book!). Weight gain during adulthood is natural, and where to draw the line between "unhealthy" weight gain and "natural" weight gain is difficult, if not impossible. In chapter four, Recognizing and Maintaining Your Natural Weight, we discuss these issues and provide a practical worksheet to determine whether weight loss is necessary. After all, the health benefits of physical activity are largely independent of changes in body weight It is very likely, however, if Americans were more physically active and actually followed this new recommendation, most U.S. adults would experience less weight gain during their adult lives.

3. To sustain weight loss in adulthood: *Participate in at least 60 to 90 minutes* of daily moderate-intensity physical activity while not exceeding caloric intake requirements. Some people may need to consult with their healthcare provider before participating in this level of activity.

   OUR TAKE: This is probably excessive, certainly for most people. The 60-to-90-minutes-per-day recommendation comes mainly from studies of men and women who have lost a substantial amount of weight, typically well over 30 pounds. For these individuals, physical activity exceeding an hour per day may be necessary to sustain such a reduced body weight. However, for the millions of people who lose more modest amounts of weight, (e.g., 5 to 20 pounds), physical activity levels of approximately 200 minutes per week of at least moderate-intensity activity are sufficient. This works out to about 30 minutes per day if performed *daily*, or about 40 to 50 minutes per day if performed *most days* (e.g., four or five days) of the week.

The *Dietary Guidelines* also provide key recommendations for specific population groups. We agree with these recommendations, and they include:

1. Children and adolescents should engage in at least 60 minutes of physical activity on most, preferably all, days of the week.

2. Pregnant women (in the absence of medical or obstetric complications) should incorporate 30 minutes or more of moderate-intensity physical activity on most, if not all, days of the week.

3. Breastfeeding women should be aware neither acute nor regular exercise adversely affects the mother's ability to successfully breastfeed.

4. Older adults should participate in regular physical activity to reduce functional declines associated with aging and to achieve the other benefits of physical activity identified for all adults.

Crawford, P., Shapiro, L., "How obesity develops: A new look at nature and nurture - Berkeley Longitudinal Studies," Obesity & Health, 3:40–41, 1991.

Johnson, S.L., Birch, L.L., "Parents' and children's adiposity and eating style," Pediatrics, 94:653–661, 1994.

Kater, K., "Real Kids Come in All Sizes: 10 Essential Lessons to Build Your Child's Body Esteem," New York, Broadway Books, 2004.

Mahan, L.K., Arlin, M., "Krause's Food, Nutrition & Diet Therapy," Philadelphia, PA, W. B. Saunders Company, 1992.

Polivy, J., "Psychological consequences of food restriction," Journal of the American Dietetic Association, 96:589–592, 1996.

Polivy, J., Herman, C., et al., Eds., "Restraint and Binge Eating. Binge Eating: Theory, Research and Treatment," New York, Springer, 1984.

Rose, H.E., Mayer, J., "Activity, calorie intake, fat storage, and the energy balance of infants," Pediatrics, 41:18–29, 1968.

Stacy, M. , "Consumed: Why American's love, hate and fear food," New York, Simon & Schuster, 1994

Ardith –
To good health!
Kurke

IT'S THE **CALORIES**,
NOT THE CARBS

The Myths and Truths of Carbohydrates

GLENN A. GAESSER, PH.D.

KARIN KRATINA, PH.D., R.D.

Note for Librarians: a cataloguing record for this book that includes Dewey Decimal Classification and US Library of Congress numbers is available from the National Library of Canada. The complete cataloguing record can be obtained from the National Library's online database at:
www.nlc-bnc.ca/amicus/index-e.html
ISBN 1-4120-3164-8

Printed in Victoria, BC, Canada

TRAFFORD

Offices in Canada, USA, Ireland, UK and Spain
This book was published *on-demand* in cooperation with Trafford Publishing. On-demand publishing is a unique process and service of making a book available for retail sale to the public taking advantage of on-demand manufacturing and Internet marketing. On-demand publishing includes promotions, retail sales, manufacturing, order fulfilment, accounting and collecting royalties on behalf of the author.
Book sales in Europe:
Trafford Publishing (UK) Ltd., Enterprise House, Wistaston Road Business Centre,
Wistaston Road, Crewe, Cheshire CW2 7RP UNITED KINGDOM
phone 01270 251 396 (local rate 0845 230 9601)
facsimile 01270 254 983; orders.uk@trafford.com
Book sales for North America and international:
Trafford Publishing, 6E–2333 Government St.,
Victoria, BC V8T 4P4 CANADA
phone 250 383 6864 (toll-free 1 888 232 4444)
fax 250 383 6804; email to orders@trafford.com

www.trafford.com/robots/04-0991.html

10 9 8 7 6 5 4 3

ABOUT THE AUTHORS

GLENN A. GAESSER, Ph.D., is a professor of exercise physiology and director of the Kinesiology Program in the Curry School of Education at the University of Virginia, in Charlottesville. Dr. Gaesser has conducted research and published many articles on exercise, body weight, health and fitness in scientific journals, trade publications, and newsletters. He is a Fellow of the American College of Sports Medicine, and co-authored this organization's 1998 position stand on "The recommended quantity and quality of exercise for developing and maintaining cardiorespiratory and muscular fitness, and flexibility in healthy adults." He is an advisory board member of, and contributing writer to, *Health at Every Size*. His interest in the relationship between body weight and health led Dr. Gaesser to author the critically acclaimed book, *Big Fat Lies: The Truth About Your Weight and Your Health*, in 1996 (updated version 2002, Gurze Books). In 1997, he received a public service award from the National Association of Anorexia Nervosa and Associated Disorders (ANAD). A popular speaker, Dr. Gaesser has presented on the subject of fitness, body weight, and health at numerous national and international meetings. He has been a guest on dozens of radio and TV shows in North America and has been interviewed for stories on body weight, fitness and health for numerous newspapers and magazines throughout the world. Dr. Gaesser has been featured on "Good Morning America," ABC's "20/20," "World News Tonight with Peter Jennings," "NBC Nightly News," CNN, and "Dateline NBC."

KARIN KRATINA, Ph.D., R.D. is a noted speaker, author, and nutrition therapist who has specialized in the treatment of weight and eating issues. She is in private practice in Gainesville, Fla. and serves as Training Consultant to The Renfrew Center, a nationally known mental health care facility specializing in the treatment of women with eating disorders. Dr. Kratina is published and frequently quoted in professional journals and the popular press. Her publications include: *Moving Away From Diets: New Ways to Heal Eating Problems and Exercise Resistance*; and chapters in *The Handbook of Medical Nutrition Therapy: The Florida Diet Manual, The Eating Disorder Sourcebook, Nutrition Therapy*, and in the upcoming eating disorders practice manual for the American Dietetic Association. She created the only interest group devoted to disordered eating within The American Dietetic Association, a group which joined SCAN (Sports and Cardiovascular Nutritionists) in 1994. Currently, she is SCAN's Chair-Elect, as well as editor for SCAN's newsletter, "PULSE." Dr. Kratina recently received the prestigious SCAN Excellence in Practice Award in Disordered Eating/Obesity.

TABLE OF CONTENTS

INTRODUCTION

FOR TODAY'S AMERICANS, it is an obsession. What should I eat? What should I avoid? Which foods should I combine? How do I get "in the zone" or "eat for my type?" We must now choose between "healthy" fats and "unhealthy" fats; "good" carbs and "bad" carbs; and "high glycemic" and "low glycemic." While the formulas for healthful eating increase, so do our waistlines.

The perfect example is the low-carbohydrate diet. Since the mid-1990s low-carb diets have made a phenomenal resurgence, led by Dr. Robert Atkins' program, which has been on *The New York Times* bestseller list continuously for the past five years. But his plan is by no means the only one. Others also are jockeying to take the low-carb crown, including the *South Beach Diet*, the latest in the low-carb offerings that has pushed its way up the bestseller lists. With this resurgence, many Americans are now avoiding carbs. For the time being, carbs appear to be the "enemy" in many people's minds and stomachs.

We emphasize "for the time being" because when it comes to diets, nothing lasts forever. Americans went through a similar obsession with carbohydrate avoidance a few decades ago, when many low-carb diet books topped the bestseller lists in the 1960s and 1970s—including the original version of Atkins' low-carb diet. Despite their popularity, low-carb diets had virtually no measurable effect on our waistlines—the weight of the average U.S. adult at the end of '70s was essentially the same as it was at the start of the previous decade. It seems that a diet limited to primarily protein and fat was not the answer after all.

The current resurgence in shunning carbs, however, is packing a lot more punch than it did during the first go-around. In fact, newspaper and magazine editors voted the resurgence of the low-carb diet as the No. 2 nutrition story of 2003. Not surprisingly, the obesity epidemic was voted No. 1, which helps explain Americans' heightened obsession with dieting. And when it comes to dieting, it seems Americans cannot resist a fad.

This time around, it seems like everyone is trying to get a piece of the low-carb action. Food manufacturers have introduced hundreds of low-carb products, which are starting to take up significant shelf space in grocery stores. Americans can now buy low-carb ice cream, beer, bread, ketchup, peanut butter, spaghetti sauce, steak sauce, and salad dressing, just to name a few. And what you cannot find in grocery stores, you can surely find on the Internet. A January 2004 search for "low-carb foods" on Google turned up more than 70,000 Web sites. Even restaurants are catering to carbohydrate phobia. T.G.I. Friday's and Subway, for example, have teamed up with Atkins. Even good ol' McDonald's is now offering low-carb meals.

The low-carb craze also is causing Americans to make some rather bizarre—and unhealthy—food choices. Sales of orange juice, for example, are down. Orange juice has never been linked to obesity or any health problem. But because it contains about 25 grams of carbohydrates per cup, orange juice has apparently become a no-no for many low-carb followers. As proof, annual consumption of orange juice has dropped by 44 million gallons since 2001. Just as alarming is the fact that from 1997 to 2003, wheat flour consumption (wheat flour is used for breads, pasta, bagels, tortillas, and other nutritious grain foods) dropped 11 pounds per person. Breads and pastas can be good sources of nutrients and whole grains, which have been associated with numerous health benefits including, ironically enough, positive weight control. In fact, some recent studies have shown high bread consumption itself to be associated with reduced risk of obesity.

How did this happen? Timing. And what might be called a collective unwillingness to examine and acknowledge the facts. Americans started getting heavier (that is, average weights started to increase) in the 1980s and 1990s, during which time "low-fat" eating became strongly encouraged. Thousands of low-fat products were introduced to the marketplace, and Americans gobbled them up. So much so that by the mid-1990s, average reported caloric intake was 100 to 200 calories per day *more* than it was in the late 1970s.

Most of the additional calories were in the form of carbohydrates. This had the effect of lowering the *percentage* of total calories coming from fat, something low-carb diet proponents have used repeatedly to bolster their claims that fat is not the problem. After all, if dietary fat intake was decreasing, fat could not possibly be the cause of Americans' expanding waistlines. Right? Well, not exactly.

Although the temporal association between Americans' increasing body weights and the increase in carbohydrate consumption during the past couple of decades is undeniable, few seem to be aware of the fact that fat consumption did *not* decrease during this so-called "low-fat" period. Quite the opposite. During the 1980s and 1990s, fat consumption (expressed in terms of grams per day, *not* as a percentage of total calories) actually *increased* slightly. The percentage went down only because fat was "diluted" by the additional carbohydrates consumed.

Truth be told, Americans never really went "low fat." It is a myth; a misnomer. The so-called "low-fat" phase of the American diet was, in reality, "high-calorie." And high-calorie generally translates to weight gain. Consuming more calories without burning them off is a recipe for obesity. **Calories—regardless of type—do count**, as Americans seem to have found out the hard way. *It's the Calories, Not the Carbs* was written in part to clarify this point and set the record straight.

It also was written to show you that eating well—and living well—is about giving yourself the best possible intake of nutrients to allow your body to be as healthy as possible and to work as well as it can. It is getting the nutrients your body needs for optimal mental performance and emotional balance. It is not a set of rules. Your body's needs and health goals are completely unique and depend on a whole host of factors—from the strengths and weaknesses you were born with, to the effects your current environment has on you. No single way of eating is perfect for everyone, although there are general guidelines that apply to us all.

Whether your personal health goal is to lose weight, maintain your current weight, become more active, have more energy, or just improve your overall health and fitness—this guide will show you how to use the Food Guide Pyramid, listen to your body, and become more active to make lasting, healthful lifestyle changes for health and wellness … and to say goodbye to fad diets of all types for good.

CHAPTER 1

The Truth About Fad Diets

IS THERE A MAGIC WAY TO LOSE WEIGHT? THIS BOOK WILL HELP YOU SEPARATE THE FACTS FROM THE HYPE.

AN ESTIMATED 50 to 70 million Americans go on diets each year. Many of these same people will go on a diet the next year. And again, the year after that. For many, this represents a cyclical pattern of yo-yo dieting that does our physical and emotional health little good. To break out of this dieting lifestyle, it is helpful to understand what you are getting into when you try to lose weight, especially if you try one of the fad weight-loss plans. First, let's test your diet IQ. Answer the following True/False questions:

1. ____ Carbohydrates are actually more fattening than fat.

2. ____ Carbohydrates are addictive and stimulate the appetite.

3. ____ Low-carbohydrate, high-protein diets are a great way to shed pounds quickly and lower your cholesterol levels.

4. ____ Weight loss is better maintained by following a low-carbohydrate, high-protein diet than it is by following a relatively high-carbohydrate, low-fat diet.

5. ____ Most popular weight-loss diets are based on sound, scientific principles.

6. ___ For optimum health and weight maintenance, foods should be eaten in certain combinations (i.e., eat foods high in protein and fat together, but eat fruits separately).

7. ___ Science tells us that carbohydrates should be divided into two groups, "good" and "bad."

8. ___ Eating fatty foods actually makes your body burn fat better and, therefore, high-fat diets are a great way to lose weight and keep it off.

9. ___ Fat is more satiating than carbohydrates.

10. ___ Assuming there are approximately 3,500 calories in one pound of body fat, eating 500 fewer calories per day (3,500 per week) will result in a loss of one pound of body weight per week, or 52 pounds of body fat in one year.

To see how you did, check your answers against the key below.

DIET IQ ANSWER KEY: ALL ARE FALSE

Below, you will find brief explanations for the answers. A more detailed look at fad diets follows in the rest of this chapter.

1. **Carbohydrates are not more fattening than fat.** In fact, the human body requires almost eight times as much energy to turn *dietary carbohydrates* into body fat as it does to convert *dietary fat* into body fat. Short-term intervention studies, as well as many large-scale population studies, show that increasing carbohydrate consumption is associated with lower body weights.

2. **Carbohydrates are not addictive, nor do they stimulate the appetite.** Some people may have cravings for certain foods, many of which contain carbohydrates. This is not addiction! Cravings are emotionally based. Complex carbohydrates are a great source of energy. They boost metabolism more than fat and are necessary to fuel a healthy body.

3. **Low-carbohydrate, high-protein diets do result in rapid weight loss, but this is largely because these diets greatly reduce the total amount of calories consumed.** As carbohydrates comprise about half of the average American diet, eliminating carbs will result in weight loss. However, most of the initial weight loss is lean tissue, not body fat. The loss of lean tissue will decrease the number of calories your body can burn, resulting in weight gain.

   Low-carbohydrate, high-protein diets do not generally lower cholesterol. Some studies reveal that these diets are more likely to raise your cholesterol levels than lower them—increasing long-term risk for cardiovascular disease.

4. **People who lose weight on low-carb, high-protein diets are about two and one-half times more likely to regain the weight than people who lose weight by following the Food Guide Pyramid's recommendations.** Also, data from the National Weight Control Registry reveal that people most successful at maintaining significant weight loss follow a diet that is relatively low in fat (20 to 25 percent) and high in carbohydrates (about 55 percent).

5. **Most popular fad diets use select-scientific principles, but taken way out of context.** A good example is the claim that carbohydrates cause insulin resistance, which leads to health

problems, including obesity. In fact, a diet high in complex carbohydrates and rich in fiber reduces your chances of developing insulin resistance. Insulin resistance is most likely to develop in people who are sedentary and eat a diet high in fat and calories and low in fiber.

6. **Contrary to the information presented in a number of popular diet books, there is no evidence that specific food combinations promote weight loss.** Total calorie intake relative to total calorie expenditure is the key. The human body does a remarkable job of absorbing the nutrients in the foods we eat, regardless of how the foods are mixed together at meals.

7. **The notion of good and bad carbohydrates is not based on sound science** and stems from the recent popularization of the glycemic index. Although the glycemic index is based on sound science, to classify carbohydrates as good or bad based solely on their glycemic index is not. All carbohydrates have nutritional value and can be part of a healthful diet.

8. **High-fat diets are not a good way to lose weight and keep it off.** Over time, eating a high-fat diet can help your body burn fat at a greater rate. The downside, however, is that you would have to consume so much fat to do this that you would actually get fatter, not thinner. A majority of scientific evidence suggests the more fat you eat in your diet, the more body fat you are likely to have.

9. **Fat is not more satiating than carbohydrates.** "Becoming satiated" refers to the process of turning off the appetite during a meal so you do not overeat. In this regard, fat has a relatively weak satiating power. Because fat has a high caloric density (nine

calories per gram vs. four calories per gram for carbohydrates and protein), eating foods high in fat increases the chances of over-consuming at meals.

10. **The arithmetic is right in terms of cutting calories, but the actual loss of body fat will rarely, if ever, match this expected result.** Cutting calories will slow your metabolism. Also, cutting calories may rob some people of energy and cause them to be less active.

FAD DIET APPEAL

Fad diets have tremendous appeal: quick, permanent weight loss; seemingly effortless; no hunger, no cravings, no calorie counting; just follow the "breakthrough" plan and the pounds just melt away; you can be thin for life. Sound familiar? For most of the last half of the 20th century, millions of Americans have tried one "breakthrough" plan after another. It is virtually impossible to go a year without some new diet plan making the bestseller lists. Since the late 1990s, diet books, at times, have regularly held half of the top-10 spots.

Despite conflicting reports about good foods and bad foods, carbohydrates vs. protein, being in the "zone" or "busting sugar," you do not need to calculate complex formulas or know what foods to combine in order to eat for well-being and enjoyment.

Our weight-obsessed culture offers the perfect environment for the gimmick-loaded diet industry. The offer of rapid and permanent weight loss sounds almost too good to be true—and, in almost all instances, it is. The trends in body weight and dieting during the past 40 years suggest that dieting may actually have an effect opposite than intended. In fact, several studies published in the past 10 years indicate that a history of dieting increases risk of future weight gain. One very recent study on school-age children revealed that dieters gained significantly more weight than non-dieters during a three-year follow-up (*Source*: Field et al., *Pediatrics*, 112:900-906, 2003.)

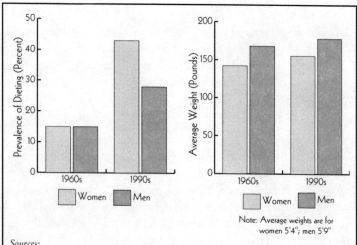

Note: Average weights are for women 5'4"; men 5'9"

Sources:

Kuczmarski, R.J., Felgal, K.M., Campbell, S.M., Johnson, C.L., "Increasing prevalence of overweight among U.S. adults. The National Health and Nutrition Examination Surveys, 1960 to 1991," *JAMA*, 272:205-211, 1994.

NIH Technology Assessment Conference Panel, "Methods for voluntary weight loss and control." *Ann. Int. Med.*, 119:760-764, 1993.

Gaesser, G.A., *Big Fat Lies: The Truth About Your Weight and Your Health*, p. 29-31, 2002.

While the prevalence of dieting has increased markedly, there has been no positive effect on our waistlines. Yet, we keep trying diets that are recycled versions of diets proven unsuccessful years earlier. The best example of this is the re-emergence of the carbohydrate-restricting diet.

CARBOHYDRATE-RESTRICTING DIETS: THE "CURRENT" RAGE

A generation ago, Americans were engaged in a similar dieting frenzy. In the 1960s and 1970s, a seemingly endless offering of low-carbohydrate diet plans was being fed to Americans just as fast as they could gobble them up. We had multi-million copy bestsellers, including *Calories Don't Count*; *The Doctor's Quick Weight Loss Diet*; *Dr. Atkins' Diet Revolution*; *The Drinking Man's Diet*; *Scarsdale*; and so on—all penned by physicians, and all urging Americans to avoid carbohydrates and eat pretty much all the fatty foods and proteins they wanted. Did we lose weight? Sure—at least for a few weeks or months. Did we keep it off? No. If any of these plans really worked, we would not have to resort to the "new" low-carb diet programs currently taking America by storm.

THE LOWDOWN ON CARBOHYDRATE-RESTRICTING DIETS

Several low-carbohydrate diet plans have made the bestseller lists: *Dr. Atkins' New Diet Revolution*; *Protein Power*; *The Zone*; *Sugar Busters!*; Suzanne Sommers' *Get Skinny on Fabulous Foods*; *The Carbohydrate Addict's Diet*; and *The South Beach Diet*, which has ranked at or near the top of virtually every bestseller list in 2003 and 2004. At the core of these diet plans is the assertion that carbohydrates make you fat.

The rationale works something like this:

Eating carbohydrates ...

	increases blood sugar
which	increases insulin secretion
which	causes excess insulin in bloodstream
which	causes an increase in hunger, making you eat more

| *and* | increases the conversion of carbohydrates into fat |
| *which* | increases body fat. |

If you consume a high-carbohydrate diet, this scenario predicts you will get fatter and fatter. But, hold on. Some parts of this rationale are fact, while others are fiction:

FACT

- Consuming carbohydrates will increase your blood sugar level—temporarily. This is a normal response to eating.

- An elevation in blood sugar will cause your pancreas to release more insulin into your bloodstream. This, too, is normal. The insulin will help to bring blood sugar back into a normal range.

- In some instances, blood sugar and insulin will increase to abnormally high levels. Foods with a high-glycemic index will result in an exaggerated increase in blood sugar and, as a result, a higher than usual increase in insulin. People who are insulin resistant generally also will have an increased insulin response, regardless of blood sugar level.

FICTION

- The exaggerated insulin response does not result in a significant conversion of carbohydrates into fat. Although many animals—pigs and cattle, for example—fatten up quite easily on carbohydrates, humans have a very poor capacity for turning carbohydrates into fat.

- It is not primarily the carbohydrates in your meal that get converted into body fat. The carbohydrates you eat are, for the most part, either burned as fuel or stored in your muscles and liver for later use. It is the *fat* in your meal that gets converted into body fat.

WHAT SCIENCE SAYS ABOUT LOW-CARBOHYDRATE DIETS

Considering the popularity of low-carb diets over the past few years, along with their popularity in the 1960s and 1970s, it is remarkable so little has been published on their efficacy. For example, until recently, only one published report on the Atkins diet had appeared in scientific literature. This study, published in the September 1980 issue of the *Journal of the American Dietetic Association*, showed that, while the Atkins diet did result in weight loss in the short term (eight weeks), it elevated total and LDL cholesterol, particularly in women. The Atkins diet also lowered HDL cholesterol in women. These results on 24 overweight men and women suggested that a low-carb diet may actually increase risk for heart disease by worsening blood lipid profile. Twenty years passed before another assessment of the Atkins diet would be published.

RECENT EVIDENCE

- In 2002, a study funded by an unrestricted grant from the Atkins Center for Complementary Medicine reported the effects of six months of very low-carbohydrate dieting on 51 overweight or obese volunteers. Only 41 completed the study. As expected with any calorie-restriction diet, participants lost weight—about 20 pounds on average. Unlike the study of the Atkins diet published 22 years earlier, total cholesterol and LDL cholesterol decreased (by 11 and 10 mg/dl, respectively), and HDL cholesterol increased (by 10 mg/dl). These reported changes in cholesterol are very much the exception with low-carbohydrate diets. Furthermore, the results are confounded by the fact that subjects were encouraged to exercise and provided nutritional supplements, including multivitamin, essential oil, and "diet" formulas designed to facilitate weight loss and improve cardiovascular risk profile. Just how much of the weight loss and changes in blood fats could be attributed to the low-carb diet itself is impossible to determine from this study. (*Source*: Westman, et al., *American Journal of Medicine*, 113:30–36, 2002).

- By contrast, another study published in 2002—not funded by Atkins—produced markedly different results with regard to health outcomes. As might be expected with any calorie-cutting diet, after one year, men and women on the low-carb diet reduced body weight (by 13.7 percent). However, their cardiovascular risk profile worsened. Total cholesterol, LDL cholesterol, and triglycerides increased, and HDL cholesterol decreased. On top of this, other blood chemicals that have been linked to vascular disease, blood clots, and stroke (homocysteine, fibrinogen, lipoprotein(a)) also increased significantly. (*Source*: Fleming, *Preventive Cardiology*, 5:110–118, 2002.)

- In 2003, results of a one-year, multi-center, randomized control trial involving 63 obese men and women were published in the May 27 issue of the *New England Journal of Medicine*. Participants on the low-carbohydrate diet lost more weight than those on a low-fat diet (25 percent of total calories from fat) during the first six months (7 percent vs. 3.2 percent), but there was no statistically significant difference in weight loss at one year (4.4 percent vs. 2.5 percent), indicating that those on the low-carbohydrate diet regained weight at a faster rate than those on the low-fat diet. Because this study did not follow subjects beyond one year, long-term efficacy of the low-carbohydrate diet could not be assessed. The authors noted that, "adherence was poor and attrition was high in both groups," adding to the already substantial body of scientific evidence questioning the wisdom of calorie-restriction practices for weight management. (*Source:* Foster, et al., *New England Journal of Medicine*, 348:2082–2090, 2003.)

- In the same issue of the *New England Journal of Medicine*, a second study reported the results of another relatively short-term (six months) study comparing a low-carbohydrate diet to low-fat diet. A total of 132 severely obese (mean BMI = 43) men and women were randomly assigned to one of the two diets. Those on the low-carbohydrate diet lost more weight (13 pounds vs. 4 pounds). Unfortunately, the study only lasted six months, which is when peak weight loss typically occurs on most diets. Had the study been extended, like the one mentioned above, the usual weight regain might have been observed. Similar to the other study, dropout rates were high in both groups. The fact that many participants were on medications (e.g., nearly one-half of the participants in the low-carbohydrate diet were on lipid-lowering drugs) further complicates the interpretation of the results. Total LDL and HDL cholesterol were not changed, although triglycerides were reduced by more in the low-carbohydrate group. (*Source:* Samaha, et al., *New England Journal of Medicine*, 348: 2074–2081, 2003.)

There are two very serious shortcomings of this study that undermine any real interpretations comparing low-carb vs. low-fat diets. First, the comparison diet, described by the authors as "low fat," was not low fat: the percentage of total calories coming from fat was 33 percent at baseline and 33 percent at six months—no change! Furthermore, the apparent weight-loss "advantage" (at least at six months) of the low-carbohydrate group cannot rightfully be attributed to a truly low-carbohydrate-type diet because the low-carbohydrate group consumed an average of 37 percent of total calories from carbohydrates during the six-month diet phase, or an average of 150 grams of carbohydrates per day (120 grams/day more than the 30 grams/day goal set by the researchers)! The real reason the "low-carb" group lost more weight was that they consumed approximately 34,000 fewer calories during the six-month period of calorie restriction (34,000 calories is almost exactly equal to the ~nine-pound difference in weight loss). And this gets to the bottom line—it's the calories, not the carbs.

FIRST-EVER SYSTEMATIC REVIEW OF LOW-CARBOHYDRATE DIETS

Yes, it is the calories! It does not matter if you cut carbs, cut fat, or a combination of both—weight loss is a matter of *amount*, not type. This has been shown in a number of very carefully controlled intervention studies. But the first thorough review of the efficacy and safety of low-carbohydrate diets was published in the April 9, 2003, issue of the *Journal of the American Medical Association*. Stanford University researchers reviewed 107 articles describing 94 different dietary interventions on a total of 3,268 participants. None of the interventions followed dieters for more than one year. Not unexpectedly, weight loss was related to diet duration and degree of calorie restriction. However, *weight loss was unrelated to reduced carbohydrate content*. Low-carbohydrate diets had no discernable effect—good or bad—on total, LDL, and HDL cholesterol; triglycerides; glucose; insulin; or blood pressure. As for weight loss, the authors concluded that, "weight loss while using low-carbohydrate diets was principally associated with decreased caloric intake and increased diet duration, but not with reduced carbohydrate content." (*Source:* Bravata, et al., *Journal of the American Medical Association*, 289:1837–1850, 2003.)

DO CARBOHYDRATES MAKE YOU FAT?

Whenever you consume more calories than you need, you will gain weight. Just how much, however, depends on a number of factors. It is much more difficult to gain weight on a diet rich in carbohydrates than it is to gain weight on a high-fat diet. The reasons for this are:

- Carbohydrates contain only four calories per gram, whereas fat contains nine calories per gram.

- Most foods naturally high in carbohydrates (e.g., grain products, foods from the base of the Food Guide Pyramid) have a low caloric density, decreasing your chance of over-consuming at meals.

In fact, data from the National Health and Nutrition Examination Survey illustrate the "nonfattening" effect of carbohydrates. In this study of a nationally representative sample of the U.S. population, dietary records of 5,730 men and 6,125 women were evaluated, along with measurements of height and weight (for calculation of body mass index, or BMI). The men and women were divided into five groups according to carbohydrate intake as a percentage of total calories. Men and women in the lowest carbohydrate intake groups consumed less than about 40 percent of total calories as carbohydrates, compared to those in the highest carbohydrate intake groups, who consumed ~60 percent or more of total calories as carbohydrates. The relationship of carbohydrate consumption to BMI can be seen in the charts on the next page.

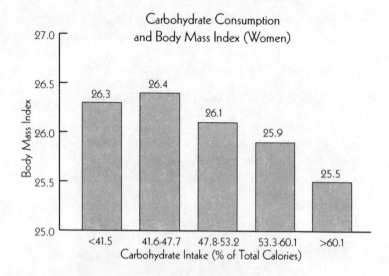

Carbohydrate Consumption
and Body Mass Index (Women)

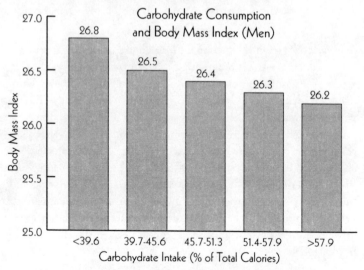

Carbohydrate Consumption
and Body Mass Index (Men)

It is quite clear from these charts that BMI actually gets *lower* as carbohydrate consumption increases, exactly *opposite* to the low-carb diet gurus' theory that carbs are making us fat. It is worth noting the striking differences between the extremes in carbohydrate consumption. Women in the highest carbohydrate intake group consume an average of 262 grams of carbohydrates per day, or about 87 grams per day *more* than women in the lowest carbohydrate intake group (175 grams per day). This works out to nearly 70 pounds *more* carbohydrate per year (87 grams per day times 365 days per year divided by 454 grams per pound) than the low-carb group—yet the "high-carb" women weigh *several pounds less* (one BMI unit is equal to about five pounds for person of average height). The same is true for men. Those in the highest carbohydrate intake group consume about 109 pounds *more* carbohydrate per year than men in the lowest carbohydrate intake—yet they, too, weigh less than their "low-carb" counterparts.

This, of course, flies in the face of the current hysteria surrounding carbohydrates and body weight. Contrary to what the low-carb diet advocates would have us believe, the results from this National Health and Nutrition Examination Survey suggest that *carbohydrates may help prevent obesity, not cause it.* This "eat-more-carbs-weigh-less" phenomenon may be due in part to the observation that, compared to lower-carb intake groups, men and women consuming the most carbohydrates consumed more fiber, less fat, and fewer total calories—all good ingredients in a healthy weight-control recipe. (*Source:* Yang, et al., *American Journal of Clinical Nutrition*, 77:1426–1433, 2003.)

This is by no means just one isolated, carb-friendly study. Results of the U.S. Department of Agriculture's (USDA) Continuing Survey of Food Intakes by Individuals, involving more than 10,000 adults, showed essentially the same thing. Men and women living on higher-carb diets, or who come closest to following the recommendations of the Food Guide Pyramid, generally weigh less than men and women consuming diets lower in carbohydrates, or who eat "non-Pyramid" diets. The authors concluded: "A study of diets of free-living adults in the United States showed that diets high in carbohydrate were both energy restrictive and nutritious and may be adopted for successful weight management." (*Sources:* Bowman and Spence, *Journal of the American College of Nutrition*, 21:268–274, 2002; Kennedy, et al., *Journal of the American Dietetic Association*, 101:411–420, 2001).

HIGH-CARBOHYDRATE INTAKE DOES NOT IMPAIR GLUCOSE AND INSULIN METABOLISM

As explained earlier in this chapter, low-carb lore tells us that carbohydrates make us fat by increasing blood sugar (glucose) and insulin, stimulating hunger to make us eat more. If this were true, we would expect blood glucose and insulin to be higher in men and women who consume the most carbs. Lore is one thing, facts are another. In the National Health and Nutrition Examination Survey study mentioned above, blood samples revealed that men and women who consume the *lowest* amount of carbohydrates have the *most* problems with insulin. The charts on the next page indicate that the low-carb groups had the highest percentage of study participants who had abnormally high insulin levels, or who had high levels of a blood protein (C-Peptide) that reflects insulin secretion rates. In other words, exactly opposite of the low-carb theory. High-carbohydrate diets, particularly those high in fiber-rich foods, tend to improve insulin metabolism, not worsen it. This explains why these very same diets *reduce*—not increase—the risk of type 2 diabetes.

Carbohydrate Consumption:
Association with High Insulin and C-Peptide (Women)

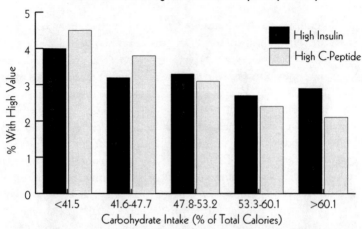

Carbohydrate Consumption:
Association with High Insulin and C-Peptide (Men)

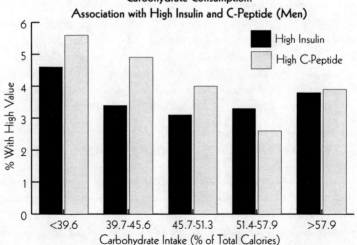

LOSING WEIGHT NATURALLY ON A HIGH-CARBOHYDRATE DIET

Not only are carbohydrates *not* fattening, a high-carbohydrate diet, especially one rich in complex carbohydrates, may actually help you lose weight naturally, without even trying. Several studies over the years have shown this to be true. One of the most recent comes from researchers in New Zealand, who examined the influence of a six-month, randomized-control dietary intervention on body weight, in which participants were asked to replace 25 percent of their normal fat intake with either 25 percent simple carbohydrates or 25 percent complex carbohydrates. Participants were not encouraged to actively reduce caloric intake, but rather replace the fat with carbohydrates.

Both "low-fat" groups averaged approximately 20 to 25 percent fat and 50 to 60 percent carbohydrate intake during the six-month intervention. Compared to the control group (30 to 35 percent fat), the "complex carbohydrate" group lost more than nine pounds during the six months—without even trying to do so. Those in the "simple carbohydrate" group did not lose weight, but they did not gain weight either (as might be predicted on the basis of current popular notions about simple carbohydrates as a major cause of obesity). Once again, the bottom line is—carbohydrates in general do not make you fat. Complex carbohydrates, in fact, may *actually help you lose weight—naturally. (Source:* Poppitt, et al., *American Journal of Clinical Nutrition,* 75:11–20, 2002.)

THE GLYCEMIC INDEX—"GOOD" AND "BAD" CARBS?

The glycemic index (GI) is a measure of how high your blood sugar rises after you consume foods containing carbohydrates. Specifically, the GI is measured by comparing the blood sugar response after consuming a specific amount of food containing 50 grams of digestible carbohydrate to that after consuming 50 grams of glucose (in some instances, white bread is used as the standard). Some carbohydrates cause your blood sugar to increase more than others. These carbohydrates are said to have a high GI. Many of the popular diet books of the past few years have labeled these as "bad" carbs.

THE FACTS

There are a number of problems with the GI. For one, the GI has a high degree of variability. For example, the 2002 International Table of Glycemic Index and Glycemic Load Values indicates the GI for carrots ranges from 16 (considered very low GI) to 92 (considered very high GI). The same table lists GIs for spaghetti ranging from 27 (relatively to low) to 65 (relatively high). Also, the GI of foods can change depending on how they are processed and prepared for consumption. Ripeness, for example, can change the GI of fruits. The way blood is sampled during a GI test can affect the result. Even within the same person, the GI can vary from one day to the next. The GI does not account for foods eaten together—as part of a meal—as foods usually are. Furthermore, ranking foods solely on the basis of GI is overly simplistic since the GI can be determined for individual foods only. Even the manner in which food is consumed can affect blood sugar response. For example, eating small meals (i.e., nibbling) throughout the day produces more stable blood sugar and insulin responses as compared to eating fewer, larger meals, even though the total amount of food—and carbohydrates—is exactly the same.

Some studies suggest that avoidance of high-GI foods may be beneficial for reducing risk of heart disease, type 2 diabetes, and certain cancers. However, the evidence is somewhat limited and inconsistent. Also, some studies show just the opposite. The Iowa Women's Health Study, for example, reported that among nearly 36,000 women tracked for six years, diabetes risk was *lower* on high-GI diets. (*Source:* Meyer, et al., *American Journal of Clinical Nutrition*, 71:921–930, 2000.) Furthermore, the American Heart Association, American Diabetes Association, and American Cancer Society do not endorse the use of the GI. In fact, no government or health professional organization in the United States endorses the use of the GI. It should be noted that, even in the studies showing an association between high-GI foods and increased risk for certain diseases, whether high-GI foods are *the actual cause*—rather than just a dietary marker for the real culprit(s)—remains to be established. Thus, at present, there is limited scientific basis for avoiding all foods that have a high GI.

GLYCEMIC LOAD: TAKING TOTAL CARBOHYDRATE CONSUMPTION INTO CONSIDERATION

The GI ranks carbohydrates in terms of blood sugar response to the consumption of 50 grams of carbohydrates. But who consumes exactly 50 grams of a particular carbohydrate at a time? To take into account not only the GI, but also the actual amount of food eaten, researchers from the Harvard School of Public Health introduced (in 1997) the concept of glycemic load (GL). Glycemic load is calculated by multiplying the GI for a given food times the number of grams of carbohydrates in one serving of that food, then dividing that number by 100. Consider the following example for four common foods that differ in GI: watermelon and pineapple, with relatively high GIs (>50), and a chocolate candy bar and chocolate cake, with relatively low GIs (<50).

Food (one serving)	GI	Carbohydrate/ Serving (g)	GL
Watermelon	75	6	4
Pineapple	59	13	7

Chocolate cake	38	52	20
Chocolate candy bar	45	28	12

Ranking solely by GI would give the impression that the chocolate candy bar and chocolate cake are superior (less fattening) to either of the two fruits. A number of other foods have high GIs but, due to relatively few calories per serving, have a fairly low GL. This again shows that ranking foods solely by GI is overly simplistic. The examples for watermelon and pineapple are particularly relevant. The *South Beach Diet* author, Dr. Arthur Agatston, lists watermelon and pineapple as the most fattening fruits, even though it would be virtually impossible to gain weight no matter how much watermelon and/or pineapple one tried to eat.

Scientifically speaking, the rationale for the GL is based on several observational studies that linked high-GL foods to increased risk for cardiovascular disease, diabetes, and certain cancers, and on a few intervention studies suggesting that a low-GL diet may be of value to persons with type 2 diabetes and as a potential obesity treatment. High-GL foods allegedly promote weight gain; however, the research is inconsistent. One large-scale study indicated that high-GL diets were associated with a slightly *lower risk* of diabetes. Another found that any deleterious impact of GL on diabetes risk could be entirely offset by increased fiber consumption. In fact, "high-GL, high-fiber" seemed to be the best combination. The link to obesity also is on shaky ground, as yet another study revealed that body weights were lowest in subjects whose diets had the highest daily GL. These findings are particularly ironic because the study was conducted by researchers from the Harvard School of Public Health, where the concept of glycemic load was developed! Although the GL may have merit in specific instances and for special populations, its practical utility for the majority of healthy adults remains to be established. Avoidance of foods like pasta, bagels, and cornflakes just because they have a high GL is not sound science.

POTENTIAL HEALTH HAZARDS OF FAD DIETING

Physical Effects

- High-protein diets may increase calcium excretion from the body and, consequently, place you at higher risk for the bone-thinning disease osteoporosis.

- Low-carb diets may increase the risk of heart disease and cancer.

- Very low-calorie dieting may deplete your body of vitamins, minerals, and essential fatty acids.

- Dieting increases risk for weight fluctuation (yo-yoing), which may increase risk for high blood pressure and cardiovascular disease.

- Rapid weight loss results in the loss of body water and lean muscle mass, not fat.

Psychological Effects

- There is potential to become apathetic, irritable, depressed, easily distracted, and less mentally alert.

- There is potential to become obsessed with food, experience intense cravings for food, and/or become possessive about food.

BREAKING THE DIET HABIT

The best way to avoid the potential hazards of nutritionally unbalanced diets is to know how to spot them. The information in this chapter should give you a good start. Just ask yourself these questions when considering a diet:

	YES	NO
Does the diet promise rapid weight loss?		
Does the diet plan rely on some miracle food?		
Does the diet plan label some foods as bad and exclude whole food groups (such as carbohydrates)?		
Does the diet plan advise supplements for everyone? Or recommend very large doses of nutrients—significantly more than 100 percent of the Recommended Dietary Allowances (RDA)?		
Does the diet plan emphasize combining foods in certain ways or avoiding certain combinations of foods (such as never eating protein with fruit)?		
Does the diet have rigid menu plans that limit food choices and does not allow you to rely on your own internal cues for hunger?		
Does the diet promise permanent weight loss with virtually no effort?		
Does the diet plan avoid the subject of exercise?		
Does the diet plan offer seemingly incredible endorsements (e.g., from celebrities), but no published scientific evidence of long-term success?		

	YES	NO
Does the diet try to lure you with scare tactics, emotional appeals, or perhaps with a "money-back guarantee" rather than proven results?		
Does the diet claim it can "treat," "cure," or "prevent" diverse health problems … from arthritis to cancer to sexual impotence?		

If the answer to any or all of these questions is yes, say no to the diet. Sound weight control advice is based on sound science.

DON'T FOLLOW THE FAD!

Before buying the latest fad diet book, take a closer look at the science behind the claims. You may be putting your health at risk without reaching your weight-loss expectations. See how these fad diets stack up against the Food Guide Pyramid. (For an in-depth book review on these diets, see Appendix C.)

Eating Plan	Premise	Missing Nutrients	Negative Health Implications	Validity	Dietary recommendations (% of total calories)
Food Guide Pyramid	The Food Guide Pyramid contains recommended ranges of all food groups, including grains, fruits and vegetables, meat, and dairy. If you follow the pyramid, you do not need to count calories or follow a strict regimen for weight management. You will get the calories and nutrients you need.	None, if the Food Guide Pyramid is used consistently	None, if the Food Guide Pyramid is used consistently	Scientific studies have proven that the most effective weight-loss program balances a healthful eating plan with regular physical activity.	50–60% carbohydrates 10–15% protein No more than 30% fat (less than 10% from saturated fat)
Sugar Busters	Sugar Busters! recommends eliminating sugar from your diet. The authors claim sugar is toxic to the body, causing the body to release insulin and store excess sugar as body fat.	Carbohydrates, vitamins, minerals	Long-term implications may include kidney and liver damage; short-term implications may include fatigue, weakness, and irritability.	Sugar Busters! is supported by testimonials of the authors' believers and anecdotal claims. Its validity is based on opinions, not proven facts.	30–35% carbohydrates from a limited food selection 25% protein 40% fat
Enter the Zone	To attain "the zone," you need to eat the proper quantities of food, in the proper macronutrient blocks" at prescribed times. This also will ensure you attain the appropriate "insulin zone."	Carbohydrates, potassium, zinc, calcium, vitamin C, beta carotene, selenium	These types of diets often lead to coronary heart disease, in addition to health problems associated with nutrient deficiencies and lack of carbohydrates.	Enter the Zone has not been validated scientifically and is supported by testimonials and poorly conducted studies.	40% carbohydrates 30% protein 30% fat (primarily from monounsaturated fats)

Eating Plan	Premise	Missing Nutrients	Negative Health Implications	Validity	Dietary recommendations (% of total calories)
Protein Power	Protein Power claims the human body has no physical need for carbohydrates, and they should be severely limited, to trick your body into burning fat without making you feel hungry.	Carbohydrates, fiber, calcium, iron, magnesium, potassium, zinc, thiamin, vitamin B6, vitamin E	The effects of a high-fat diet may include increased risk for coronary heart disease, high cholesterol, liver and kidney damage, some cancers, and osteoporosis.	The authors claim success through testimonial anecdotes and book sales. No scientifically validated studies suggest that the Protein Power diet works.	15% carbohydrates 25% protein 60% fat
Dr. Atkins' New Diet Revolution	The book suggests drastically reducing the intake of dietary carbohydrates to force your body to burn your reserve of stored fat for energy. This will result in losing pounds and inches, while still eating protein and fat-laden foods.	Carbohydrates, calcium, magnesium, potassium, iron, thiamin, vitamin C, vitamin E	Increased risk of cardiovascular disease, high cholesterol, liver and kidney damage, some cancers, and osteoporosis.	There are no scientific studies to show this diet works in the long term. Recent short-term studies suggest that it may not adversely affect cholesterol.	15% carbohydrates 30% protein 55% fat
The Heller's Carbohydrate Addicts Lifespan Program	An excess of insulin, the "hunger hormone" causes the carbohydrate addict to experience intense and recurring cravings, as well as the heightened ability to store fat. The affected person has a biological condition caused by a hormonal imbalance which can be corrected by following their program.	Carbohydrates, vitamins, minerals, fiber	These types of diets often lead to coronary heart disease, in addition to health problems associated with nutrient deficiencies and lack of carbohydrates. Short-term implications may include fatigue, weakness, and irritability.	No success-rate data or case studies are published anywhere in the book or a scientific journal. Success is demonstrated by personal testimonials, anecdotes from the Hellers' patients, or the Hellers' personal success stories.	15–35% carbohydrates 24–40% protein 45–70% fat

Eating Plan	Premise	Missing Nutrients	Negative Health Implications	Validity	Dietary recommendations (% of total calories)
Dr. Bob Arnot's Revolutionary Weight Control Program	Foods are drugs. Eating certain foods will make you feel terrible and gain weight, while other foods will guarantee weight loss. Arnot promotes a "feedforward" eating plan which will teach you in what order and at what times of day to eat foods to maximally control your weight, hunger, and mood.	Carbohydrates, vitamins, minerals	Health problems associated with nutrient deficiencies and lack of carbohydrates.	There have been no scientifically validated studies conducted on Dr. Arnot's eating plan. Arnot's "validation" for his book comes from his friends and relatives.	55–65% carbohydrates (from limited food selections) 20–25% protein 15–20% fat
The South Beach Diet	The latest of the low-carb diets. The first two weeks of total carbohydrate avoidance results in rapid weight loss. Carbohydrates are divided into "good" and "bad." The book blames the USDA Food Guide Pyramid for the "fattening of America."	Carbohydrates, vitamins, minerals	Low-carb diets such as this may increase risk for cardiovascular disease, in addition to health problems associated with nutrient deficiencies and lack of carbohydrates.	No peer-reviewed studies of this diet have been published. Efficacy is based solely on testimonials. It is estimated that less than 10% of Americans follow the Food Guide Pyramid, yet nearly two-thirds are considered overweight or obese.	20–30% carbohydrates 20–30% protein 45–50% fat
The Ultimate Weight Solution	A behavior-change weight-loss program — with no recipes! Diet success is dependent on seven keys to weight-loss freedom." Based on a lot of common sense.	Carbohydrates	Potential health problems associated with low intake of whole grains.	No peer-reviewed studies of this weight-loss plan have been published. If Dr. Phil follows his own plan, it is probably safe to say it does not work — he is 35 pounds overweight!	40–50% carbohydrates 20–30% protein 20–30% fat

THE SOUTH BEACH DIET

BY ARTHUR AGATSTON, M.D.

WHAT THIS DIET IS ABOUT

This is the latest of the low-carb diets. Carbohydrates are classified as "good" and "bad" on the basis of their glycemic index. Dr. Agatston blames Americans' weight problems on the USDA Food Guide Pyramid: "The best intentions of the USDA and its pyramid turned out to be a diet based on sugars. It is the widespread adoption of this way of thinking that has caused the fattening of America."

PLUSES

- Dr. Agatston advocates dietary fiber, and his recommendations for carbohydrate consumption beyond the initial two-week, highly restrictive Phase 1 are not as severe as other low-carbohydrate plans.

- Dr. Agatston criticizes other low-carbohydrate plans, such as Atkins, that allow virtually unlimited consumption of foods high in saturated fat.

PITFALLS

- The 14-day, Phase 1 period is extremely restrictive: absolutely no bread, pasta, potatoes, rice, or fruit. No alcohol of any kind. No sugar, candy, cake, cookies, or ice cream. He claims you will lose eight to 13 pounds in the first two weeks. By cutting out all carbohydrates, which comprise about 50 percent of the calories consumed by the average American, it is not hard to see why.

- Most of the initial weight loss on low-carb diets is water.

- Phase 2 (which continues "until you hit your target weight") and Phase 3 (maintenance) are described in less than 250 words each!

- The book relies exclusively on anecdotal testimonies. There is no published evidence this diet is sustainable and will result in permanent weight loss.

- Carbohydrates are rated on the basis of their glycemic index. According to Dr. Agatston's charts, watermelon is more fattening than a chocolate candy bar, pretzels are a sure-fire ticket to obesity, and a baked potato is practically the worst thing you could eat. In fact, Dr. Agatston asserts that, "a baked potato will be less fattening with a dollop of low-fat cheese or sour cream." Even though the potato with the dollop of low-fat cheese or sour cream has more calories, Dr. Agatston claims it will be less fattening because the fat slows down digestion. To the contrary, research has shown that when fat (such as in cheese or sour cream) is added to a high-carbohydrate meal, it is the added dietary fat—not the carbohydrates—that is converted to body fat.

- Dr. Agatston also claims, "French fries are better than baked, because of the fat in which they are cooked." French fries are high in total fat and loaded with trans fats. No reputable nutritionist would recommend french fries over a baked potato.

THE ULTIMATE WEIGHT SOLUTION

by Phil McGraw, Ph.D.

What this diet is about

This weight-loss plan relies on what Dr. Phil refers to as "seven keys to weight-loss freedom": 1) Right thinking (unlocks the door to self-control); 2) Healing feelings (unlocks the door to emotional control); 3) A no-fail environment (unlocks the door to external control); 4) Mastery over food and impulse eating (unlocks the door to habit control); 5) High-response cost, high-yield nutrition (unlocks the door to food control); 6) Intentional exercise (unlocks the door to body control); and 7) Circle of support (unlocks the door to social control).

Pluses

- Exercise is one of the seven keys. Research has shown regular exercise is vital for long-term weight control and maintenance of weight loss.

- Dr. Phil advocates fiber-rich foods, which are important for health and long-term weight control. He encourages the reader to stock the kitchen with fruits, vegetables, whole grains, lean meats, low-fat products, and sugar-free beverages.

- With the exception of the recommendation for carbohydrates (only two to three servings a day), the dietary recommendations are very similar to that of the USDA's Food Guide Pyramid: two servings of fruit, four servings of vegetables, three servings of protein, two servings of low-fat dairy products; and one serving of fat (emphasis on monounsaturated fats, fish, nuts, and seeds).

- Dr. Phil's recommendations for estimating portion sizes, and how to divide up the plate at mealtime to emphasize plant-based foods, is commendable.

- Dr. Phil at least mentions size diversity, acknowledging the genetic reality that bodies come in a variety of shapes.

PITFALLS

- This is a behavioral change weight-loss plan, and it is doubtful the average reader will have the skills to incorporate all of the recommendations.

- Dr. Phil's body weight recommendations are much stricter for women than they are for men. According to "Dr. Phil's Body Weight Standards," the upper limit for women for body weight corresponds to a body mass index (BMI) of about 25. For men, the upper limit for body weight corresponds to a BMI of 29 to 30. Dr. Phil does not explain his reasons for this, but it may have something to do with the fact that at 6'4" and 240 pounds (BMI = 29+), Dr. Phil is considered severely overweight by current U.S. government guidelines. Of course, one way to not be overweight is to just change the guidelines!

- Dr. Phil asserts all overweight individuals are malnourished ("If you are overweight then, by definition, I know you are malnourished"). This is a ridiculous statement. There is no evidence to support such a categorical statement about large individuals. In fact, his assertion seems entirely inconsistent with his acknowledgement that, "God brought us into this world in a pleasing array of diverse shapes and sizes, and we are genetically programmed to be a certain way: tall, short, muscular, stout, or thin as a fiddle string." Dr. Phil claims to "know the science," but there is little evidence to indicate he knows much of anything about obesity.

- Dr. Phil claims an 80 percent success rate (for individuals losing 100 to 300 pounds), yet provides no evidence for this. Even with structured weight-loss programs involving nutritionists and counselors, long-term efficacy of behavioral interventions is poor.

- Adopting Dr. Phil's recommendations for "high-response cost foods" ("those that require a great deal of work and effort to prepare and eat") may be easier said than done. Most people "know" they should eat more fruits, vegetables, and whole grains, but few actually do.

ENTER THE ZONE

BY BARRY SEARS, PH.D.

WHAT THIS DIET IS ABOUT

The "zone" is a state where the mind is relaxed and focused and the body is fluid and strong. Sears believes insulin is the cause of weight gain, so people must attain the appropriate insulin "zone."

PLUSES

- Sears believes it is a good idea to drink water, exercise, and snack throughout the day.

- Sears realizes some fat is necessary in the diet.

PITFALLS

- You will need to eat rigid quantities of food at prescribed times, with EXACTLY 40 percent of calories from carbohydrates, 30 percent from fat, and 30 percent from protein at every single meal and snack. With a fast-paced lifestyle, the last thing you may want to do is follow a strict, controlled eating regimen—particularly when eating can and should be a pleasurable experience.

- Hope you like math. You will have to calculate your protein requirements based on several tables and complex charts. You also will need to follow the "macronutrient block method" for determining when and how many "blocks" to eat each day. Maintaining these rules permanently may be hard to do—even for the most dedicated and loyal follower.

- Sears recommends eating very few calories. Specifically, 500 calories or less at any one meal and 100 or less for snacks. Some menus on Sears' diet call for fewer than 800 calories per day. As long as you can adhere to such strict guidelines, you will probably lose weight—as well as enjoyment of food. Any low-calorie recommendation may be dangerous and should be medically supervised.

- You will need to eliminate certain carbohydrates (your body's fuel food), such as pasta, bananas, breakfast cereals, potatoes, breads, sandwiches, and carrots. Unfortunately, these foods include vitamins and minerals your body needs, are a great source of energy, and are typically low in fat. The Sears' eating plan also is typically low in calcium, which may set you up for osteoporosis down the line.

PROTEIN POWER

BY MICHAEL R. EADES, M.D., AND MARY DAN EADES, M.D

WHAT THIS DIET IS ABOUT

If you cut carbohydrates to "make room" for extra protein and fat, your body will be tricked into burning fat without making you feel hungry. Food is used to "condition" your body, and fat is a high-octane energy source.

PLUSES

* The Eades recommend exercising and drinking a lot of water.

PITFALLS

* To comply with this diet, you will have to design your meals based on lists of specific foods and guidelines that vary depending on whether you are in the "Intervention," "Transition," or "Maintenance" level of the program, and whether you opt for the "Hedonist," "Dilettante," or "Purist" approach. You may have a hard time maintaining these rules permanently, even if you are a dedicated and loyal follower. The last thing you may want to do is follow a strict, controlled eating regimen—particularly when eating can and should be a pleasurable experience.

* Unfortunately, you will need to cut out carbohydrates—your body's fuel food—no matter in which level of the program you are. Fruits, vegetables, and grain foods are typically low in fat, include essential vitamins and minerals your body needs, and are a necessary energy source for your body.

* Many of the *Protein Power* meal choices amount to eating very few total calories per day. As long as you can adhere to such strict

guidelines, you will probably lose weight—as well as enjoyment of food.

- Any low-calorie recommendation may be dangerous and should be medically supervised.

DR. BOB ARNOT'S REVOLUTIONARY WEIGHT CONTROL PROGRAM

BY ROBERT ARNOT, M.D.

WHAT THIS DIET IS ABOUT

Arnot believes that foods are drugs. Eating certain foods will make you feel terrible and gain weight, while other foods will guarantee weight loss. The book proposes to alter your body's physiology from weight gain to weight loss—and maximally control your weight, hunger, and mood—by eating foods in a certain order and at certain times of the day.

PLUSES

- Arnot promotes eating fiber as a healthful weight-loss tool.

PITFALLS

- You will need to restrict high-glycemic index foods, such as bananas, carrots, potatoes, white bread, bagels, pasta, and muffins. Unfortunately, these foods provide essential vitamins and minerals your body needs, are a great source of energy, and are typically low in fat. Avoiding these foods, without reason, will make you miss out on important nutrients.

- To comply with the diet, you will need to design your meals based on "Feedforward Eating," which will teach you in what order and at what times of day to eat. The day is divided into zones (The Power Zone, The Loading Zone, The Craving Zone, The Relaxation Zone, The Fat Zone, and The Workout Zone), each of which is complete with multiple meals from which you can pick and choose. You may have a hard time maintaining these rules permanently, even if you are a dedicated and loyal follower.

- Eating should not be this hard. The last thing you may want to do is follow a strict, controlled eating regimen—particularly when eating can and should be a pleasurable experience.

THE CARBOHYDRATE ADDICT'S LIFESPAN PROGRAM: A PERSONALIZED PLAN FOR BECOMING SLIM, FIT, AND HEALTHY IN YOUR 40S, 50S, 60S, AND BEYOND

BY RICHARD F. HELLER, M.S., PH.D., AND
RACHAEL F. HELLER, M.A., M.PH., PH.D.

WHAT THIS DIET IS ABOUT

An excess of the "hunger hormone" insulin will cause you (the carbohydrate addict) to experience intense and recurring food cravings, as well as the heightened ability to store fat. A carbohydrate addict has a biological condition caused by a hormonal imbalance, which can be corrected by following the "STAR Program"— **S**imple, **T**argeted to one's needs and decade of life, **A**daptable to one's lifestyle, and a program that **R**ewards a person with food they love.

PLUSES

- The Hellers condemn prejudice toward people who are overweight.

- They realize some carbohydrate-rich foods are needed for "energy, nutrition, and satisfaction" and allow all foods to be included in the diet somewhere.

- They stress the importance of choosing a realistic weight goal based on your age, body build, and health needs, and recommend a reasonable weight loss of one-half to two pounds a week.

PITFALLS

- To comply with this diet, you will need to make sure to get equal portions of carbohydrate, protein, and fat at your "Reward Meal," which must be eaten in the span of one hour. If you have seconds, you must have seconds of everything. You may have a hard time maintaining these rules permanently, even if you are a dedicated and loyal follower.

- Eating should not be this hard. The last thing you may want to do is follow a strict, controlled eating regimen—particularly when eating can and should be a pleasurable experience.

- Where's the exercise? A person who exercises will reap health benefits independent of weight loss!

- The Hellers believe you do not need breakfast. In fact, breakfast is essential for health and weight loss/maintenance! It gives you a head start on getting nutrients your body needs.

- Where is the fiber? It is highly unlikely the diet will allow you to consume the recommended 20 to 35 grams of fiber per day—a proven key in weight control.

- The plan sets you up for disappointment. You must weigh yourself each day and record your weight on the Progress Chart to gauge your average weekly weight loss. However, for some people, weight can fluctuate from three to five pounds a day or naturally vary by several pounds. You are better off focusing on healthy eating habits rather than daily weight.

DR. ATKINS' NEW DIET REVOLUTION

BY ROBERT C. ATKINS, M.D.

WHAT THIS DIET IS ABOUT

Atkins believes there is one basic factor that controls obesity—insulin. He promises you can still lose pounds and inches while you eat as many, or even more, calories than you might normally, from predominantly protein and fat-laden foods. The one requirement is you must drastically reduce your intake of dietary carbohydrate, thus forcing the body to burn your reserve of stored fat for energy.

PLUSES

• A full chapter is devoted to the benefits of exercise.

• Atkins suggests everyone have a medical checkup to determine general health status before starting the diet.

PITFALLS

• The diet is unbalanced and excessively high in protein and fat, especially saturated fat (unlimited consumption of meat, eggs, and cheese is recommended), which can increase your risk of developing heart disease and some cancers.

• Atkins advises against consuming carbohydrates (your body's main fuel) such as breads, cereals, fruit, starchy vegetables, and milk. Limiting these foods will mean you are limiting vitamins (thiamin, niacin, and folic acid), minerals (calcium), antioxidants, and fiber you get from fruits, vegetables, and whole grains.

• The diet does not allow you to eat any sugar and/or refined carbohydrates. In fact, no food is bad for your health, when eaten in moderation. All foods can fit into a healthy diet.

- Dr. Atkins promises fast and significant weight loss. In reality, successful and safe weight loss does not happen overnight, or even in a week or two. It requires a great deal of effort and a commitment to healthy lifestyle changes.

- Dr. Atkins advocates purchasing several supplement pills—primarily his own. Not only is this expensive, but also unnecessary. A balanced diet that incorporates a wide variety of foods will give your body the nutrients it needs.

- No bones about it, your body will have a hard time absorbing minerals such as calcium on this diet, potentially putting you at greater risk of developing osteoporosis. The diet also may lead to dehydration and, over time, place excessive demands on your kidneys and liver.

- Without carbohydrates, your body cannot burn fat efficiently, allowing "ketones" to accumulate in the blood. This leads to "ketosis"—a condition often accompanied by nausea, headaches, fatigue, and bad breath—and signals that the body is in a starvation state.

SUGAR BUSTERS!

BY H. LEIGHTON STEWARD, MORRISON C. BETHEA, M.D.,
SAM S. ANDREWS, M.D., AND LUIS A. BALART, M.D.

WHAT THIS DIET IS ABOUT

Eating sugar causes the body to release insulin, a hormone that promotes fat storage, resulting in obesity from an "insulin overload." According to the authors, decreasing sugar intake can help you trim body fat and lose weight, regardless of whatever else you eat.

PLUSES

- The diet allows whole grains and some vegetables. You will get some great sources of fiber, vitamins A and C, some B vitamins, and zinc.

PITFALLS

- All white potatoes/rice/bread, refined sugar, corn syrup, molasses, honey, sugared colas, corn, carrots, and beets are considered the enemy and severely restricted. In fact, no food is bad for your health. By listening to your internal cues, any and all foods can fit into a healthy diet. This advice ignores the nutritional value, vitamins, and minerals many of these foods contribute to the diet—such as calcium, folic acid, and iron.

- You may get obsessed with every gram of sugar—unnecessarily.

- There are many strict rules to follow. Fruit should always be eaten by itself, and you will need to avoid eating high glycemic index carbohydrates and fats at the same meal, if possible. You may have a hard time maintaining these and other rules permanently, even if you are a dedicated and loyal follower.

- Eating should not be this hard. The last thing you may want to do is follow a strict, controlled eating regimen—particularly when eating can and should be a pleasurable experience.

- Pass on the water, as well as the bread. On the *Sugar Busters!* eating plan, you must only drink fluids in small quantities during meals. The truth is, consuming enough fluids is important for maintaining and regulating balance, preventing headaches and fatigue associated with dehydration, and helping with weight loss.

CHAPTER 2

Using the Food Guide Pyramid

WHAT YOU EAT CAN MAKE A BIG DIFFERENCE TO YOUR HEALTH. JUST REMEMBER,
WHAT COUNTS IS PROGRESS, NOT PERFECTION.

WHETHER YOU WANT to lose weight or just be healthier, the key is to make small changes one step at a time that lead to a long-term lifestyle change in the way you look at eating and exercise.

Whether you have made lowering fat or eliminating the so-called "bad" carbs in your diet the ultimate quest, it is easy to forget the big picture—that healthful eating means eating a variety of foods, *including* breads, other grain foods, fruits, vegetables, and so on. Enjoy a wide variety of foods you like, and take time to listen to your body's internal cues to tell you when, what, and how much to eat.

WHAT IS THE FOOD GUIDE PYRAMID?

"I want to lose weight," you say, "but I just don't know what to do. Losing weight and eating foods for specific nutrient benefits seems way too complicated. One day you hear a food is good for you, the next day it is bad. I'm so confused!" Many fad diet gurus have taken advantage of this nutrition information (and misinformation) overload and have preyed on consumers' desire for a magic bullet solution, often suggesting consumers eliminate entire food groups that provide many nutrients our bodies need. Unfortunately, there isn't a magic formula for every meal of the day, and eliminating entire food groups and the benefits they provide causes more problems than solutions.

But there is a guide that can help you on your road to healthier eating. With the Food Guide Pyramid, developed by the USDA and recognized by well-known nutrition authorities, you can focus on listening to your own internal cues and do not need to obsess about your food choices. The Food Guide Pyramid:

- Is flexible and easy for everyone to use. You do not have to learn a new system for eating or cross any foods off your list.

- Recognizes that rigid food rules are nearly impossible to follow, at least for the long term, because they take the fun out of a social activity all of us want to enjoy … eating! By focusing on what to include in our daily meals rather than what to avoid, the Food Guide Pyramid can help take some of the stress out of eating well.

- Includes variety, balance, and moderation. The Food Guide Pyramid gives you a guideline as to how much food to eat to get all the nutrients your body needs.

- Includes foods from all cultures. No matter what your cultural heritage is, your traditional foods will fit. In fact, the Food Guide Pyramid has gone global, with a number of countries having developed their own versions. Although subtle differences exist, the core recommendations are basically the same: A big thumb's up to grains, fruits, vegetables, lean meats, and low-fat dairy products; go sparingly on sweets, added sugar, and fats.

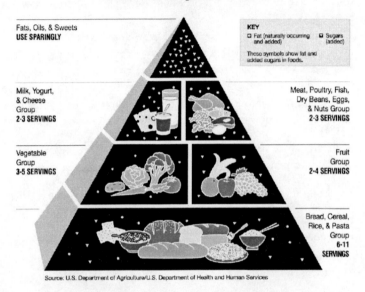

Food Guide Pyramid
A Guide to Daily Food Choices

Fats, Oils, & Sweets
USE SPARINGLY

KEY
□ Fat (naturally occurring and added)   ▣ Sugars (added)
These symbols show fat and added sugars in foods.

Milk, Yogurt, & Cheese Group
2-3 SERVINGS

Meat, Poultry, Fish, Dry Beans, Eggs, & Nuts Group
2-3 SERVINGS

Vegetable Group
3-5 SERVINGS

Fruit Group
2-4 SERVINGS

Bread, Cereal, Rice, & Pasta Group
6-11 SERVINGS

Source: U.S. Department of Agriculture/U.S. Department of Health and Human Services

One of the biggest benefits of the Food Guide Pyramid is that it focuses on eating normally: eating for health and enjoyment. The definition of "normal" eating emphasizes the importance of listening to our own internal cues to help us decide what and how much to eat. Many people lose the ability to eat normally when they diet or attempt to manipulate their food choices.

FOOD GUIDE PYRAMID UNDER ATTACK

During the past few years, the USDA's Food Guide Pyramid, with grain-based foods at its base, has come under attack. Criticism has come mainly from low-carb diet advocates, but also from some health professionals who blame the Food Guide Pyramid as one of the contributing causes of America's obesity problem. One prominent researcher from the Harvard School of Public Health asserted in the January 19, 2004, issue of *Newsweek* that the USDA Food Guide Pyramid was "poorly built" and that Dr. Atkins was "at least half right in condemning carbohydrates." According to pyramid critics, the carb-rich foods at the base are a recipe for weight gain and the diseases frequently associated with obesity, such as diabetes and heart disease.

Actually, the pyramid was researched and built on a scientific base. And, before condemning carbs, consider this:

- Large-scale studies indicate that body weights are lowest for men and women consuming *high*-carbohydrate diets.

- Long-term weight loss and maintenance is better on relatively high-carb diets.

- High-carbohydrate diets tend to have the highest diet quality and are associated with reduced risk of a number of degenerative diseases, including cardiovascular disease and diabetes.

As for the claim that the pyramid has contributed to America's obesity problem, that is a case of very fuzzy math. Approximately two-thirds of U.S. adults are considered overweight or obese. By contrast, less than one in ten Americans actually follows the recommendations of the Food Guide Pyramid. How can you blame a weight-gain problem affecting 65 percent of the population on something that less than 10 percent actually follow? It does not add up.

And neither do the assertions of the pyramid attackers. In reality, if more of us really did follow the recommendations of the pyramid, we might be *slimmer* for our efforts. Persons who follow a pyramid-based diet are more likely to have body weights in the normal range.

ALTERNATIVE VERSIONS OF THE PYRAMID

Several alternatives to the USDA Food Guide Pyramid have been proposed. A vegetarian alternative, for example, with more food groups, has been developed for persons who choose to avoid some, or all, animal products. Other than placing water (8 cups per day) at the base and the absence of all animal products except dairy products (for lactovegetarians), the rest of the pyramid is generally the same as the USDA version.

A Mediterranean Food Pyramid, with more emphasis on monounsaturated fats, such as olive oil, has also been proposed. Grains, fruits, and vegetables are still featured prominently near the base, along with legumes and nuts. The biggest difference is the placement of meat at the tip with the recommendation to consume "monthly."

The most recent challenge to the USDA's version is the Healthy Eating Pyramid developed by Dr. Walter Willett and his colleagues at the Harvard School of Public Health. Major differences include:

1. Adding daily exercise and weight control to the very base of the pyramid.

2. Placing plant oils next to whole grains near the base of the pyramid, just above exercise and weight control.

3. Making a separate category for vegetable protein (nuts and legumes) in the middle of the pyramid, right below animal sources of protein (poultry, fish, and eggs).

4. Placing refined grains (white bread, rice, pasta, and potatoes) at the tip of the pyramid, along with sweets, red meat, and butter.

How does this alternative rate? First of all, the USDA is in favor of exercise and weight control, so there really is no disagreement with emphasizing exercise and weight control.

Making a separate, more dominant category for vegetable sources of protein is not a bad idea. Nuts and legumes are great sources of protein, and both foods have been shown in many studies to be linked to better health and reduced risk of several diseases. This distinction may be more appealing to vegetarians.

However, by placing vegetable oils near the base of the pyramid, the Healthy Eating Pyramid may make it more difficult to maintain a healthy weight. After all, fats—regardless of source—contain 9 calories per gram, twice as many as carbohydrates and protein.

And restricting consumption of white bread and rice, potatoes, and pasta! There is no consistent or compelling evidence to show that severely restricting consumption of these foods is a good thing. Many studies show that potatoes and pasta, as well as white bread and rice, are totally compatible with good health and weight control. The recommendation to "use sparingly" is based on the notion that these foods contain a lot of refined carbohydrates—the so-called "bad" carbs.

"BAD" CARBS ARE GETTING A BAD RAP

Carb critics do not condemn all carbs, only those they refer to as the "bad" carbs, such as highly processed, refined grains and sugar. Refined grains, critics claim, are essentially the same as sugar, and are to blame for obesity and health problems associated with excess weight, such as heart disease and diabetes. Because the USDA Food Guide Pyramid does not distinguish between highly processed and minimally processed (whole) grains, critics contend that the USDA's pyramid could lead to health problems in persons whose servings from the bread, cereal, rice, and pasta group come mainly from refined grains rather than whole grains.

It is true that whole grains have been shown to have greater overall health benefits than their refined counterparts because of the higher fiber and phytonutrient levels. But that does not mean that refined grains have no place in our diet. Condemning refined grains as inherently "bad" is not justified. Actually, the results of several studies reveal a not-so-bad-after-all picture of refined grains. For example:

- Results from the latest (third) National Health and Nutrition Examination Survey indicate that high consumption of carbohydrates, even refined carbohydrates, is associated with *lower* body weights, not higher. Rather than contribute to obesity, carbs (even refined ones) may actually help prevent it.

- Among the nearly 36,000 women participating in the Iowa Women's Health Study, consumption of high-glycemic foods (so-called "bad" carbs) was not associated with increased risk of diabetes. In fact, women who consumed the most "bad" carbs actually had slightly *lower* risk of diabetes than women who consumed the least amount of these high-glycemic foods.

- Similar to the findings from the Iowa women, a recent study of several thousand middle-aged men and women in Finland revealed that refined grain consumption was associated with *reduced* risk of diabetes, not an increased risk.

And do not forget that refined grains are fortified with folic acid—twice as much folic acid as can be found in whole grains. According to the Centers for Disease Control, neural tube defects (NTD), debilitating birth defects, have decreased by 23 percent following folic acid fortification of grain foods. In March 2004, the Centers for Disease Control (CDC) released a paper reporting that, since folic acid fortification to enriched grains was mandated in 1998, there have been 31,000 fewer stroke-associated deaths and 17,000 fewer deaths related to ischemic heart disease in the U.S. *each* year. Preliminary research also indicates folate's probable value in preventing some cancers, as well as improving memory.

Our point here is that labeling foods—in this case carbs—as either "good" or bad" is not based on sound science. Making an effort to choose more foods rich in whole-grains is wise, especially considering that Americans average less than one serving of whole grains per day. But elimination of refined grains is neither necessary nor justified. All foods can fit in a healthy diet. And as for weight control, again we must emphasize that it's the calories, not the carbs.

MAKING THE BEST OF THE CURRENT VERSION OF THE USDA FOOD GUIDE PYRAMID

In general, the basic structure of the current pyramid is fine. However, a lot of research since its introduction in 1992 suggests that it might be wise to think about the following when making choices:

1. Choose at least three whole grain options daily, particularly emphasizing high-fiber alternatives. But also remember that refined grains provide health benefits, too, and can be a healthy food choice.

2. Limit consumption of saturated and trans fats (discussed in chapter 3) found in many processed foods; for example, replace butter and regular margarine with "trans fat-free" alternatives.

3. Choose low-fat versions from the traditional protein sources (such as low- or non-fat dairy products, fish, poultry, and lean meat) along with vegetable sources of protein (such as legumes and nuts).

HOW TO USE THE FOOD GUIDE PYRAMID

All sections of the Food Guide Pyramid are important. However, foods from the wide "base" area of the pyramid are designed to be the "base" of your diet. So, aim to select a majority of food from the bottom half—grains, fruits, and vegetables. The pyramid also breaks down each food group into ranges of servings, so it is easier to see how much food you need daily to provide your body with the nutrients it needs.

For most people, understanding what amount of food constitutes a serving may be a little challenging. We will talk about serving sizes for all the food groups a little later, but in the meantime, remember this: you need to know what a serving is to get the nutrients your body needs.

FOOD GUIDE PYRAMID GROUP	SERVINGS
Bread, Cereal, Rice, and Pasta	6-11
Vegetables	3-5
Fruit	2-4
Meat, Poultry, Fish, Dry Beans, Eggs, and Nuts	2-3
Milk, Yogurt, and Cheese	2-3
Fats, Oils, and Sweets	Use sparingly

How many servings within each range should I strive for?

The chart below suggests more specific guidelines for how many Food Guide Pyramid servings to choose daily (based on gender and activity level), if you select mostly low-fat and lean foods with moderate amounts of fats, oils, and sweets.

	Less Active Women, Older Adults	Children, Teen Girls, Active Women, Less Active Men	Teen Boys, Active Men
Calories	About 1,600	About 2,200	About 2,800
Grains Group	6*	9*	11*
Vegetable Group	3	4	5
Fruit Group	2	3	4
Milk Group	2-3**	2-3**	2-3**
Meat Group	2, for a total of 5 ounces	2, for a total of 6 ounces	2, for a total of 7 ounces

*Strive for at least three of these servings from whole grain foods.
**Women who are pregnant or breast-feeding, teenagers, and young adults to age 24 need three servings.

To help you remember these recommendations, place a photocopy of the pyramid on your refrigerator. It is an excellent visual reminder of the basics of a healthful diet, so every time you walk to your fridge, take a look. Where are you in terms of the range of servings—what your body needs—from each food group for the day?

If you are concerned about your weight, do not shy away from the pyramid! Even eating the upper range of recommended servings from each group may result in weight loss for many active people.

Do I need to measure servings?

No. Use servings only as a general guide. For "mixed" foods, do the best you can to estimate the food group servings of the main ingredients. For example, a serving of pizza might count in the grain group (crust), the milk group (cheese), and the vegetable group (tomato sauce, any vegetable toppings). A helping of beef stew would count in the meat group and the vegetable group. Both have some fat—fat in the cheese on the pizza and in the gravy from the stew, depending on how it is made. The USDA allows dry beans, peas, and lentils to be counted in the meat group or counted as servings of vegetables—but not both.

A LOOK AT THE FOOD GROUPS IDENTIFIED IN THE FOOD GUIDE PYRAMID

Bread, Cereal, Rice, And Pasta Group

6–11 Servings Per Day

What counts as a serving?
- 1 slice of bread
- 1 oz. or 1/2 cup of ready-to-eat cereal
- 1/2 cup of cooked cereal, rice, or pasta
- 1 tortilla (6" diameter)
- 6 saltine crackers
- 1/2 bagel or English muffin

Feel free to enjoy oversized bagels you can buy at a bakery or a plate of pasta from an Italian restaurant—just remember that they can count as 2 to 5 servings from this group.

What's in it for me?

Grain foods play an important role in our diets by providing a wide array of nutrients.

Grain foods are nutrition powerhouses that provide:
- Complex carbohydrates
- Vitamins and minerals (including folic acid)
- Phytonutrients and antioxidants
- Fiber

Most foods from this group are cholesterol-free, naturally low in fat and sodium, and an excellent source of energy your body needs on a daily basis. Contrary to what diet "experts" say, grain foods are a key part of any diet which helps you maintain or achieve a healthy weight.

Enriched and fortified grains are a good source of folic acid, as well as other necessary B vitamins and iron. Whole grain and enriched grain foods provide a concentrated source of natural antioxidants, which are thought to protect against heart disease and cancer. Whole grains also are an excellent source of phytoestrogens, which may protect against breast and prostate cancer, and fiber—typically containing 2 or more grams per serving.

The National Academy of Sciences recommends that adults less than 50 years of age eat 25 to 38 grams of fiber (with women at the lower end of the scale and men at the higher end) each day for good health, yet most of us barely eat half that amount. In order to get the fiber your body needs, strive for three whole grain servings per day. How to find whole grains? Check the ingredient list to see if the first ingredient listed is a whole grain such as "whole grain wheat," "whole wheat," or "whole wheat flour."

HOW DO I ADD GRAINS TO MY DIET?

- Rearrange your plate. Give grains the spotlight and plan the rest of the meal around them.

- Keep a "grains stash" handy to help curb those midday hunger pangs. Keep a bag of low-fat grain snacks nearby, such as pretzels, graham crackers, or your favorite cereal.

- Go international. Besides the usual rice and pasta, try "ethnic" grains such as quinoa, amaranth, bulgur, couscous, barley, oats, buckwheat, and rye, which have a lot to offer in terms of taste, texture, and nutrition.

- Mix different types of pastas together, such as whole grain, spinach, and regular pasta.

- Add some crunch to your soup, salad, or yogurt. Sprinkle granola, wheat germ, or crushed, flaked cereal on top.

- Have a sandwich—the official meal to go—by using different types of breads, from white, rye, and whole wheat, to tortillas for wraps and pitas for handy pocket sandwiches.

THE GOODNESS OF WHOLE GRAINS

Although whole grain foods are loaded with fiber, they are a great source of other health-enhancing compounds as well.

- Antioxidants, thought to protect against heart disease and cancer.

- Resistant starch, thought to play a complementary role to fiber in the prevention of some bowel diseases, reduction of blood cholesterol levels, and control of blood glucose.

- Phytoestrogens, thought to protect against breast and prostate cancers, and also may help with menopausal symptoms.

- Magnesium, now thought to play a vital role in maintaining healthy glucose metabolism.

- Vitamin E, which has been reported to be associated with reduced risk of diabetes.

- Vitamin B_6 and folic acid, which may help lower blood levels of homocysteine, now considered a risk factor for heart disease, stroke, and diabetes; folic acid also may help reduce risk of Alzheimer's disease and childhood leukemia.

- Other phytochemicals, which may play a wide range of roles in preventing chronic disease.

PUTTING RESEARCH INTO PRACTICE

Many studies have proven the goodness of whole grains. For example, a number of large-scale studies have reported associations between whole grain consumption and reduced risk of heart disease and diabetes. But what exactly does that mean? How much do I need to make sure I get enough?

Actually, getting the most out of whole grains is not all that hard or time consuming. For starters, just one additional serving per day will do wonders. Consider the following:

- In many studies, the maximum benefit of whole grains is seen with adding just one serving of whole grains per day. In one study of 86,000 male physicians, those who consumed at least one serving per day of whole grain breakfast cereal had a 20 percent lower risk of cardiovascular disease, compared to men who rarely consumed breakfast cereal. Even men who consumed *only a few servings per week* had an 18 percent lower risk. So it does not take much to get the benefit.

- Similarly, data from the Nurses' Health Study show that an increase in cereal fiber intake of just 5 grams/day might reduce the risk of coronary heart disease in women by 37 percent. This amount of fiber can be found in a bowl of cereal (see tables of fiber-rich foods).

- In a study of more than 50,000 health professionals, increasing cereal fiber intake by just 1.4 grams per day more than the "high-risk" group that consumed only an average of 2.7 grams per day, reduced risk of peripheral arterial disease by 31 percent. A small bowl of cereal or a bran muffin will have at least that much fiber. Interestingly, in this study upping cereal fiber intake to more than 10 grams per day was not associated with any further risk reduction. Once again, small changes can lead to big benefits.

- Benefits also come fast. Within a matter of weeks, sometimes even days, increased whole grain consumption improves insulin and glucose control, and lowers cholesterol and blood pressure.

- It is never too late! A recent study of older men and women revealed that cereal fiber consumption was inversely related to cardiovascular disease. For example, the amount of cereal fiber contained in just two slices of whole grain bread was associated with a 14 percent lower risk of cardiovascular disease.

Because the evidence is so strong, the U.S. Food and Drug Administration (FDA) approved the following health claim that allows food companies to promote the heart disease and cancer-fighting benefits of whole grains: "Diets rich in whole grain foods and other plant foods, and low in total fat, saturated fat, and cholesterol may reduce the risk of heart disease and certain cancers."

Despite the goodness of whole grains and this endorsement by the FDA, Americans do not consume enough of them, falling well short of the recommended three servings per day. In fact, only about 8 percent of U.S. adults consume three servings per day. Most Americans average less than one serving per day; 20 percent of adults and 40 percent of children never eat whole grains!

As the studies mentioned above show, something as simple as adding a whole grain serving is all it takes. Or, you could try a whole grain breakfast cereal a few times per week, and a whole grain muffin or English muffin on the other days. Actually, breakfast is a great way to start out the day with whole grains. A recent study showed that eating cereal for breakfast was associated with significantly lower body weight as compared to eating meats and/or eggs, or skipping breakfast altogether.

REMEMBER, ENRICHED GRAINS ARE GOOD TOO!

The current *Dietary Guidelines for Americans* recommends that consumers "choose a variety of grains, especially whole grains." Although we have emphasized the importance of whole grains, enriched grains should not be viewed as "poor" choices. Enriched grains have health benefits as well. White bread, for example, made from enriched flour, is a good source of iron and B vitamins, and can contain as many antioxidants as a number of fruits and vegetables.

Enriched grains are "enriched" with iron, folic acid, niacin, thiamin, and riboflavin. Over the years, enrichment has helped eliminate many diseases caused by deficiencies in these nutrients, such as beriberi, pellagra, and severe iron anemia. Folic acid enrichment has greatly reduced incidence of neural tube birth defects (see chapter 2). Folic acid enrichment also has had other positive health benefits. For example, a 2004 study showed for the first time that folic acid intake was associated with decreased risk for ischemic stroke in more than 40,000 men participating in the Health Professional Follow-Up Study.

FINDING THE FIBER

Many grain foods are good sources of fiber. Listed below are a few examples.

EXAMPLES OF GRAIN-BASED FOODS	FIBER (GRAMS)
1 oz. (3/4 cup ready-to-eat cereal)—bran, oat, wheat flakes	2-9
1/2 cup whole wheat noodles, cooked	3-4
1/2 cup whole wheat pasta	6
1 English muffin	2
1 slice whole wheat bread	2-3
1 slice white bread	.5
1 (6" diameter) pita bread, white	1-2
1 (6" diameter) pita bread, whole wheat	3-4
1/2 cup spaghetti or macaroni, cooked	.5
1/2 cup rice, cooked	.5-2
6 whole wheat crackers	2-3
6 saltine crackers	1
1 tortilla (6" diameter)	1-2
1/2 cup flour, all-purpose (white)	2
1/2 cup flour, whole wheat	6-7

FRUIT GROUP

2–4 Servings Per Day

WHAT COUNTS AS A SERVING?

- 1 medium piece of fresh fruit
- 1/2 cup of chopped, cooked, or canned fruit

- 3/4 cup of fruit juice

Aim to get at least the absolute minimum of two servings a day. Although you do not have to choose two different fruits, variety is always a good idea. Let yourself enjoy more if you are still hungry.

VEGETABLE GROUP
3–5 Servings Per Day

WHAT COUNTS AS A SERVING?
- 1 cup of raw leafy vegetables
- 1/2 cup cooked vegetables
- 3/4 cup vegetable juice

Aim to get at least the absolute minimum of three servings a day. Although you do not have to choose three different vegetables, variety is always a good idea. Again, let yourself enjoy more if you are still hungry.

WHAT'S IN IT FOR ME?

These foods are usually low in calories and, similar to grains, play an important role in our diets with their wide array of nutrients. Unfortunately, national surveys show that fewer than 15 percent of Americans eat even the minimum five servings of fruits and vegetables a day. Fruits and vegetables are nutrition powerhouses that give your body:
- Vitamins A, C, and beta carotene
- Minerals such as iron, magnesium, and potassium
- Fiber
- Phytochemicals

Like grains, fruits and vegetables also are naturally low in calories, fat, and sodium, and are cholesterol-free. That is why it is best to get a majority of your nutrients and calories from the bottom portion of the pyramid. And consider this: fruits and vegetables with the deepest colors are the richest in antioxidants and phytonutrients, which may help prevent many types of cancer.

HOW DO I ADD FRUITS AND VEGETABLES TO MY DIET?

Let yourself enjoy more than the 5-a-day minimum if you are hungry. They are great in-between-meal snacks, whether you are working at your desk, driving the kids to soccer practice, or reaching for an after-dinner treat. Try these suggestions for adding more to your meals. Remember, eating any fruit or vegetable—whether fresh, canned, or frozen—is an improvement over not eating any at all. Begin with the fruits and vegetables you do like.

- Always have fresh fruits and veggies ready to eat. Chop ahead of time and store in the refrigerator for instant eating. Ready-to-use produce, such as bagged, fresh spinach and baby carrots, makes it easy to add vegetables liberally to recipes.

- Grow a vegetable garden. There is nothing like the flavor of a homegrown vegetable, and kids love them. If space is limited, try planting in a pot.

- Use fruits to accent foods whenever possible. Top cereals, pancakes, desserts, and yogurt with pieces of fruit.

- Puree a vegetable and add it to a sauce or soup.

- Keep skins of fruits and veggies on when possible to get the most fiber (and take advantage of the convenience!). Remember to scrub well—using water and a vegetable scrub brush.

- Use frozen fruit in milkshakes. Or make your own simple fruit "slush" by blending fresh sliced fruit with ice.

- Disguise a vegetable. Snipped ribbons of spinach and other leafy greens resemble herbs such as basil.

- Keep dried fruit on hand in a convenient place—like your brief-case, desk drawer, or glove compartment—for a quick snack, or when you are low on fresh fruit.

- Ask grandma to teach you how to make those collard, mustard, and other greens that have been the favorites of southerners for generations.

- Suspend fruit—in gelatin, that is—for a refreshing, appealing fruit snack.

MILK, YOGURT, AND CHEESE GROUP
2–3 Servings Per Day

Aim for an absolute minimum of two calcium-rich servings from this group each day. Teenagers, young adults to age 24, and women who are pregnant or breastfeeding, should aim for a minimum of three servings.

WHAT COUNTS AS A SERVING?

    1 cup of milk or yogurt
    1-1/2 oz. of natural cheese
    2 oz. of processed cheese

WHAT'S IN IT FOR ME?

    Vital nutrients that dairy foods provide include:
- Minerals such as calcium, phosphorous, and magnesium
- Riboflavin (vitamin B_2)
- Protein

Calcium is an important mineral for men and women, and getting enough makes a difference at any age. Many promising studies show that calcium not only helps maintain bone health, but also reduces colon cancer risk, decreases risk for kidney stones, and helps prevent high blood pressure during pregnancy. Calcium also has been shown to help with weight reduction.

Many dairy foods are excellent sources of calcium. Listed below are a few examples.

DAIRY PRODUCT	CALCIUM (Milligrams)
1 cup fat-free milk with nonfat milk solids	316
1 cup skim milk	300
1 cup 2% milk	295
1 cup 1% low-fat milk	295
1 cup buttermilk	285
1 cup yogurt (low-fat)	420
1 cup yogurt (non-fat)	450
1 oz. mozzarella cheese, part-skim	185
1 oz. cheddar cheese	205
1/2 cup cottage cheese	75

Other foods also supply calcium, such as deep-green leafy vegetables and fish with edible bones. Many processed foods, such as soy milk, orange juice, breakfast cereal, and even some breads, may be fortified with calcium as well.

How do I add dairy foods to my diet?

Although the Food Guide Pyramid recommends two to three servings each day, most teenagers and women get barely half that amount. Try these tips to get the servings of dairy foods your body needs, and kick up the calcium in your diet:

• Enjoy yogurt with your meals or as a quick, easy snack. Low- and non-fat varieties are available.

• When preparing oatmeal or other hot cereals, make them with low-fat milk.

- Get your just desserts! Puddings are an excellent source of milk and can be made with skim or low-fat milk.

- Have a tasty breakfast beverage. Mix milk, calcium-fortified orange juice, and a banana.

- Add some pizza pizzazz to your meals. Not only is pizza a great source of calcium, but also an opportunity to add vegetable toppings.

- Use milk as a substitute for water when making soup, or add nonfat, dried, powdered milk to oatmeal, soups, and casseroles.

- Opt for lower-fat versions, such as low-fat chocolate milk or cocoa—get the same chocolate satisfaction but with less fat.

- If you are not that fond of the taste of milk, try adding vanilla, almond, or coconut extract to change the flavor.

- Say cheese please. Sprinkle cheeses on salads, side dishes, or casseroles.

Meat, Poultry, Fish, Dry Beans, Eggs, And Nuts Group
2–3 Servings Per Day

What counts as a serving?
- 2-3 oz. of cooked lean meat, poultry, or fish—about the size of a deck of cards or the palm of your hand.
- 1/2 cup of cooked dry beans, 1 egg, or 2 Tbsp. of peanut butter equal 1 ounce of meat.

What's in it for me?
- Protein
- B vitamins such as folic acid and vitamin B_{12}
- Minerals such as iron, potassium, and zinc

- Fiber (only from beans and nuts)

How do I add protein to my diet?

If you are like many Americans, the challenge may not be getting enough meat or protein in your diet—but not overdoing it. Take another look at the Food Guide Pyramid. The size of the meat group is fairly small in comparison with grain foods, fruits, or vegetables.

The key is to focus on reducing the fat while keeping the flavor and the iron. That said, do not be afraid to include lean red meat in your diet. Many have sworn off red meat in the interest of low-fat eating. As a result, iron intake has decreased—especially in women of childbearing age. Even a marginal iron deficiency can affect your energy level and interfere with your ability to perform at your full potential. Make the most out of the iron in grain foods by "partnering" them with vitamin C-rich foods at a meal—the iron absorbed by your body will be boosted by two- to four-fold.

Here are some suggestions to raise your iron while keeping fat intake low:

- Try fish for a lean entrée—it has both iron and a type of protein that enhances iron absorption.

- Add green bell pepper (high vitamin C) to a lean roast beef sandwich or in your favorite chili.

- Choose lean cuts of red meat, pork, and poultry without skin. Top round steak is the leanest cut of beef and a great source of iron.

- Throw some toasted pumpkin or sesame seeds on a chicken salad made with spinach greens. The iron from the chicken and vitamin C from the spinach will increase the iron absorption from the seeds.

- Bake, broil, boil, or grill your steak, hamburger, pork chops, chicken, or fish instead of frying.

- Crisp it up—try a three-layer coating for meats. First dip in flour, then in an egg white wash, and then add a crunchy coating like cornflake crumbs.

- In the mood for a burger? Grill the burger (letting the excess fat drip), then blot on paper towels to remove additional fat.

Although beans—dried beans, peas, or legumes such as lentils and pinto beans—are often overlooked as part of the "meat" group—they are not only low in fat, but also high in protein, fiber, and folic acid. Studies continue to highlight the role of beans in reducing risk of heart disease and certain cancers, decreasing cholesterol, and keeping blood sugar levels more stable (an advantage for people with diabetes). You also may want to consider adding nuts and seeds to main/side dishes—they are higher in fat and calories, but contain "heart healthy" types of fat.

Try these tips:

- Add kidney beans, garbanzo beans, or sunflower seeds to your salad.

- Toss some black beans into a taco with the usual toppings.

- Try using tofu in recipes. Add it to pasta dishes like lasagna or soups.

- Try an easy beginner's step and purchase the ready-to-make bean soups that come with an assortment of beans and seasonings. All you do is provide the water.

- Try a chili bean pita. Fill pita bread with your favorite chili beans, top with low-fat cheddar cheese, and heat in the microwave until melted.

- Order a bean burrito at a fast food restaurant.

FATS, OILS, AND SWEETS
Use sparingly

WHAT COUNTS AS A SERVING?

Although not a "food group"—with no recommended range of daily servings—fats, oils, and sweets are located at the tip-top, and smallest part, of the pyramid. Likewise, your body needs few foods that are comprised mostly of fats, oils, and sweets—such as cream, butter, margarine, soft drinks, candies, and sweet desserts—for good health.

Let's say that one day you have cheesecake for breakfast, lunch, and dinner. You even have it for a snack in between meals. Check in with your body. How do you feel? Chances are you are getting some kind of feedback. Chances are your body will be craving the nutrients you are missing from not eating any foods from the other groups of the Food Guide Pyramid. You may get negative feedback from your body and feel uncomfortable or sluggish. Although this may be an extreme example, the point is a good one to remember.

WHAT'S IN IT FOR ME?

Contrary to popular belief, fat is not all bad. Your body needs fat from food to:

- Help your body absorb and transport some vitamins (A, D, E, and K)

- Provide your body with energy to fuel your physical activity

- Build brain and nerve tissues, and body cell walls

Your body needs stored fat to:

- Maintain body heat

- Protect your vital organs

- Build an energy reserve

Besides these things, fat helps make food taste and smell good. Fat also plays a role in satisfying hunger—giving you a feeling of fullness and minimizing between-meal hunger pangs. However, evidence is clear that a diet high in fat, especially saturated fat, relates to many chronic health problems; among them, heart disease, some types of cancer, diabetes, and obesity. The American Heart Association, American Cancer Institute, and the USDA/DHHS (United States Department of Agriculture/Department of Health and Human Services) Dietary Guidelines for Americans recommend Americans limit fat in their diets to 30 percent of total daily calories (67 grams of fat for a 2,000 calorie diet). You could get up to half this amount even if you pick lower fat choices from each food group and add no extra fat to your foods during preparation or at the table.

How do I limit fat in my diet?

Try the three suggestions below for cutting fat in your diet:

- Discover how you can cut the fat without missing it or feeling deprived. Rather than trying to take the fat out of all your recipes, try one fat-cutting technique at a time and build on your success.

- When possible, choose healthier fats. The healthiest fats are low in saturated fat. Examples include canola, corn, olive, safflower, and sunflower oil.

- When you eat fat, make sure to enjoy it, and do not feel guilty! It is okay to want to taste every gram.

But beware: low-fat may not mean low-calorie. You must be careful not to misinterpret that "fat-free" also means "calorie-free." To find out if a "fat-free" food also is a high-calorie food, you must read the Nutrition Facts label. Fat-free or reduced-fat products may be just as high—or higher—in calories than the regular version. Here are a few examples:

Fat-free/Reduced-fat Product	Calories	Regular Product	Calories
Reduced-fat peanut butter (2 Tbsp.)	190	Regular peanut butter (2 Tbsp.)	190
Reduced-fat chocolate chip cookie	128	Regular chocolate chip cookie	136
Fat-free fig cookie	70	Regular fig cookie	50
Non-fat frozen yogurt (1/2 cup)	190	Regular ice cream (1/2 cup)	180
Reduced-fat ice cream (1/2 cup)	190	Regular ice cream (1/2 cup)	180
Reduced-fat granola cereal (1/4 cup)	110	Granola cereal (1/4 cup)	130
Baked tortilla chips (1 oz.)	110	Regular tortilla chips (1 oz.)	130

SERVING SIZES—A CHEAT SHEET

Snacks and meals eaten away from home may provide a large part of the nutrients your body needs. So, it helps to know how many servings of a food you are eating. If you have trouble visualizing what a serving size looks like, it may be helpful to refer to the examples below to estimate your portions:

- 3 ounces of meat is about the size and thickness of a deck of playing cards or an audiotape cassette.

- A medium apple or peach is about the size of a tennis ball.

- 1 ounce of cheese is about the size of 4 stacked dice.

- 1/2 cup of ice cream is about the size of a racquetball or tennis ball.

- 1 cup of mashed potatoes or broccoli is about the size of your fist.

- 1 teaspoon of butter or peanut butter is about the size of the tip of your thumb.

- 1 ounce of nuts or small candies equals one handful.

Sometimes, you may choose to eat only a fraction of what is on your plate, but other times, you may decide your body needs "the whole thing" to keep your diet healthful and nutritious.

CHAPTER THREE

Nutrients—The Building Blocks of Good Health

WHAT NUTRIENTS DOES YOUR BODY NEED FOR HEALTH AND WELLNESS? THIS
CHAPTER WILL HELP YOU UNDERSTAND THE VALUE OF NUTRIENTS IN FOOD.

THE SCIENCE BEHIND good nutrition is complex, and getting the nutrients
your body needs every day for good health can seem like a daunting
task. The human body requires 55 nutrients for proper growth and
health, including macronutrients (protein, fat, and carbohydrates),
micronutrients (vitamins and minerals), and water.

It would be very difficult to track your intake of 55 nutrients every
day. That is why the Food Guide Pyramid was developed—to provide
a personal guide for making healthful food choices. Individual foods
vary in the types and amounts of nutrients they provide, so if you
choose a variety of foods daily from each of the Food Guide Pyramid
groups, an adequate intake of these 55 nutrients is virtually assured.

Think of food as little packages of nutrients! Each food group provides some, but not all, of the nutrients you need each day. That means
that foods in one group cannot replace those in another. No single
nutrient is most important—for good health, you need them all.

In this chapter, the focus is on protein, carbohydrates, and fat, because the foods in which they are found provide virtually all of the
vitamins and minerals we need, as well as the calories to keep our
bodies going.

PROTEIN

Protein was the first substance to be recognized as a critical component of the body. Its name was derived from the Greek word *protos*, which means "first."

WHAT IS PROTEIN?

Protein is often referred to as a single nutrient. Yet, in reality, protein is composed of 20 building blocks, known as amino acids. Nine of these amino acids cannot be made by your body, so you must get them from the foods you eat. They are called essential amino acids.

WHAT IS PROTEIN USED FOR?

Protein is used by your body in many ways, among which are:

- Building and maintaining muscle and other body tissues

- Providing an energy source when carbohydrates are not available

- Making enzymes and hormones

- Maintaining a healthy immune system

WHAT ARE GOOD PROTEIN SOURCES?

Animal sources like dairy products, meat, eggs, poultry, and fish, as well as soy products and various beans and legumes, are excellent sources of protein. Although almost every food of plant origin (fruits, vegetables, grain foods) contains some protein, it is a much smaller amount.

HOW MUCH PROTEIN DO YOU NEED?

Most of us get plenty of protein in our diets, so it is not a nutrient that we should be concerned about. If you follow the Food Guide Pyramid, you will naturally get about 10 to 15 percent of your total daily calories from protein. Most adults in the United States average closer to 15 percent. However, people who try to lose weight on low-calorie diets may not get enough protein.

CARBOHYDRATES

Think of carbohydrates as gas in your fuel tank. Without them, you simply will not have the energy to function. These sugars and starches are your body's main source of fuel, powering everything from jogging to breathing, and even to digesting food. Carbohydrates in foods come in two main types: simple and complex.

SIMPLE

Simple sugars are classified as either monosaccharides ("mono" meaning one, and "saccharide" meaning sugar) or disaccharides, which are two monosaccharide sugar molecules joined together ("di" meaning two). Frequently referred to as sugars, or simple sugars, these are quite common in the American diet. Some examples are:

- Sucrose (table sugar), a disaccharide made up of glucose and fructose

- Lactose (sugar found in milk), a disaccharide made up of glucose and galactose

- Fructose (sugar found in fruit and honey), a monosaccharide

Natural or refined sweeteners, such as corn syrup, maple syrup, high-fructose corn syrup, honey, molasses, and fruit juice concentrate, also are simple carbohydrates.

Glucose is the most common simple sugar and is present in all disaccharides. Glucose also is the form of carbohydrate that the body uses for energy. Regardless of the type ingested, all carbohydrates are ultimately converted to glucose so the body can use them as fuels.

Complex

Carbohydrates consisting of more than two sugar molecules are called complex carbohydrates. These can come in relatively short carbohydrate "chains" of between three and 10 sugar molecules (called oligosaccharides—"oligo" meaning scant or few) or very long carbohydrate chains containing hundreds, sometimes thousands, of sugar molecules, called polysaccharides ("poly" meaning many). Polysaccharides come in two basic types: starch (digestible) and fiber (indigestible). (More on fiber later.)

Carbohydrate-rich foods are terrific sources of vitamins and minerals, and many are great sources of fiber. Some examples are:

- Grain foods (e.g., bread, cereal, and pasta), which make up the base of the Food Guide Pyramid, *including both enriched and whole grains*

- Vegetables (e.g., potatoes, peas, and beans)

How are carbohydrates used?

- **To prime metabolism.** Your body needs adequate carbohydrates to be able to burn fat—as often said, "Fat burns in a carbohydrate fire."

- **As a key source of fuel** for muscles and the brain.

- **To fuel your body** during vigorous, high-intensity exercise.

- **To prevent excessive breakdown** of muscle and other body protein for energy.

- **To protect your body** from a condition called ketosis, with symptoms of weakness, nausea, and dehydration.

- **To help normal fat metabolism.** When there is a lack of carbohydrate, more fat is used for energy than the body is equipped to handle, which may lead to dehydration.

HOW MUCH CARBOHYDRATE DO YOU NEED?

The Food Guide Pyramid is an excellent visual reminder of the importance of carbohydrates as the basis of a healthy diet with the foundation as the Breads, Cereals, Rice, and Pasta Group. According to a 2002 report from the National Academy of Sciences' Institute of Medicine, it is a good idea to make carbohydrates—particularly complex carbohydrates—provide at least half of your total daily calories. It is recommended that 45 to 65 percent of your calories be in the form of carbohydrates.

For your health, make foods rich in complex carbohydrates your body's main energy source. Not only are they a great way to get the vitamins and minerals you need, but many are a great source of fiber as well. An added bonus: most of these foods also are relatively low in total and saturated fat.

SIMPLE OR COMPLEX ... DOES IT MATTER?

In terms of energy, no. Whether simple or complex, all carbohydrates provide four calories of energy per gram—the same as protein. However, with regard to health and weight control, complex carbohydrates—largely due to their fiber content—are preferred. But this does not mean you need to completely avoid simple carbohydrates. Both simple and complex carbohydrates can fit into a healthy diet.

Consumption of simple carbohydrates has increased dramatically during the past few decades, mostly in the form of sweeteners such as high-fructose corn syrup. High intake of simple sugars has frequently been blamed for a host of health problems, including obesity. However, the bulk of scientific evidence does not support a cause and effect link. For example, high sugar consumption is not associated with higher body weight, nor is sugar consumption necessarily associated with poor glucose control, diabetes, cardiovascular disease, or hyperactivity in children. In fact, the only health problem that sugar consumption has been convincingly linked to is dental caries. But do not take this to mean that once you have passed your cavity-prone years, unlimited consumption of sugar is a good thing.

Although the optimum amount of sugars in the diet is not known, 25 percent of total calories consumed is maximal intake level. Higher amounts may be associated with reduced intake of important micronutrients (i.e., the "empty calorie" effect of consuming foods composed primarily of added sugars). For example, approximately one-third of total added sugar consumption in the United States is in the form of soft drinks. And, because the increased consumption of added sugars has contributed to the increase in total calorie consumption during the past few decades, cutting back on consumption of soft drinks and similarly sweetened drinks is probably not a bad idea.

In contrast to simple carbohydrates, consumption of fiber-rich complex carbohydrates has not increased in the past few decades. This is unfortunate because consumption of complex carbohydrates is associated with lower risk of diabetes, heart disease, gastrointestinal disorders, certain cancers, and obesity. The critical health-enhancing ingredient in complex carbohydrates is fiber.

FIBER—THE "UNSUNG" NUTRIENT

Fiber comes from a wide variety of whole grain products and fruits and vegetables, including legumes (e.g., beans and peas). Consuming more complex carbohydrates by following the Food Guide Pyramid will help you get the fiber your body needs.

There are many studies that attest to the health benefits of fiber. Take a look:

- Helps lower blood cholesterol and may reduce risk of death from heart disease.

- Helps play a role in preventing and treating diabetes by improving blood sugar control and increasing sensitivity to insulin.

- May help protect against colon cancer.

- Helps protect against other bowel disorders, such as constipation, hemorrhoids, and diverticulosis.

- Helps with weight control. You may feel more satisfied and eat less at subsequent meals.

FILLING YOUR MEALS WITH FIBER

Try these tips to help you get the fiber your body needs:

- When baking breads, cookies, muffins, or brownies, try using ⅓ to ½ whole wheat flour in place of all-purpose flour.

- Buy whole grain bread and crackers. Be sure the first ingredient is whole wheat flour or a type of whole grain.

- Crumble graham crackers with wheat germ and cinnamon. Sprinkle over applesauce for an afternoon snack.

- Munch on low-fat popcorn for a satisfying whole grain snack.

- Choose whole grain and high-fiber cereals that can provide more fiber per serving.

- For a convenient breakfast, buy frozen whole grain waffles. Just pop into the toaster.

- Top whole wheat pita bread with pizza sauce, mozzarella cheese, and a dash of oregano. Heat in the microwave until melted for a quick pita pizza snack.

Source: Evelyn Tribole, M.S., R.D., Stealth Health, 1998

THE FIBER FACTOR

If you are wondering how much fiber you are getting from the foods you eat, take a look at the list below.

Food/Amount	Fiber (grams)
Breads, grains, and pasta	
Bagel, 1 medium	1
Breadstick, 1	<1
Noodles, ½ cup	1
Brown rice, cooked, ½ cup	2
French bread, 1 slice	<1
Pumpernickel bread, 1 slice	3
Spaghetti, cooked, ½ cup	1
Wheat bran, 1 Tbsp.	2
Wheat germ, 1 Tbsp.	1
White bread, 1 slice	<1
White rice, cooked, ½ cup	1
Whole wheat bread, 1 slice	2
Whole wheat pasta, ½ cup	6
Breakfast cereals	
100 percent bran, ⅓ cup	8
Bran flakes, ¾ cup	5
Corn flakes, ¾ cup	1
Granola w/raisins, ¼ cup	2
Oatmeal, cooked, ¾ cup	3
Raisin bran, ¾ cup	5
Shredded wheat, 1 cup	6

Food/Amount	Fiber (grams)
Fruits	
Apple, w/skin, 1 medium	3
Applesauce, ½ cup	2
Apricots, dried, 12 halves	4
Banana, 1 medium	2
Blackberries, ½ cup	3
Blueberries, ½ cup	2
Figs, dried, 2	4
Orange, 1 medium	3
Pear, w/skin, 1 medium	4
Prunes, dried, 3	2
Raisins, ¼ cup	2
Raspberries, ½ cup	4
Strawberries, 1 cup	4
Vegetables, cooked	
Broccoli, ½ cup	2
Brussels sprouts, ½ cup	3
Peas, ½ cup	2
Potato, baked, w/skin, 1 medium	4
Potato, mashed, ½ cup	1
Spinach, ½ cup	2
Sweet potato, baked, w/skin, ½ medium	2
Vegetables, raw	
Carrots, 1 medium	2
Lettuce, romaine, 1 cup	1
Spinach, 1 cup	1
Tomato, 1 medium	2

Food/Amount	Fiber (grams)
Beans, cooked	
Baked beans, ½ cup	6
Kidney beans, ½ cup	6
Lentils, ½ cup	8
Refried beans, ½ cup	6
Snack foods and nuts	
Almonds, ¼ cup	3
Bagel chips, 5 pieces	4
Hummus dip, 2 Tbsp.	2
Macadamia nuts, ¼ cup	3
Peanuts, dry-roasted, ¼ cup	3
Pecans, ¼ cup	3
Popcorn, air-popped, 1 cup	1
Sunflower seeds, ¼ cup	4
Trail mix, ½ cup	4
Walnuts, ¼ cup	2

*All values are rounded. Due to the different methods used to determine fiber in foods and to "round" values, the grams of fiber listed on Nutrition Facts panels and in other sources may differ slightly from those listed above.

Sources: Bowes and Church's Food Values of Portions Commonly Used, 16th Edition, 1994; Plant Fiber in Foods, 2nd Edition, 1990; and manufacturer data, adapted from The American Dietetic Association's Complete Food and Nutrition Guide, 1998.

ACHIEVING YOUR FIBER GOAL

The recommended daily intake of fiber is 25 to 38 grams. Most Americans consume only about one-half of this amount. This is primarily due to inadequate consumption of fruits, vegetables, and whole grain products. Following the Food Guide Pyramid can help you achieve this goal. Most grain servings will have at least 1 to 2 grams of fiber per serving. Most fruits and vegetables will have 2 to 3 grams of fiber per serving. So just meeting the minimum recommendation for servings of fruits and vegetables, and from foods at the base of the pyramid, will give you approximately 20 grams of fiber per day. If you make an effort to eat just one very high-fiber food per day, such as a bowl of high-fiber breakfast cereal or a cup of bean soup, along with your regular servings of fruits, vegetables, and other grain products, this should put you well over the 25-gram-per-day minimum.

For example, see how eating the following foods during a typical day can help boost your fiber intake.

Food	Fiber (grams)
Breakfast	
Raisin bran cereal, ¾ cup	5
Orange, 1 medium	3
Lunch	
Sandwich, with whole grain bread	4
Salad, lettuce with ½ tomato and croutons	2
Snack	
Trail mix, ½ cup	4
Dinner	
Spaghetti, 1½ cups	3
Carrots, equivalents to 2 medium	4
Applesauce, ½ cup	2
Total for the day	27

Remember, the health benefits of fiber are greatest when increasing from the level in the typical American diet to the minimum recommendation of 25 to 38 grams per day. So just adding one or two fiber-rich foods to your diet—even if you change nothing else!—can have a big impact on your health. One recent study indicated that each 5-gram-per-day increase in fiber consumption reduced the risk of heart disease by over 20 percent! You can find that much fiber in just one bowl of cereal (see table above).

FOLIC ACID—THE OTHER "UNSUNG" NUTRIENT

Folic acid, or folate, is a B vitamin important for red blood cell and nervous system development. The best benefit of folic acid is its role in decreasing risk of neural tube birth defects, such as spina bifida. Recent research also has shown that folic acid may reduce the risk of cardiovascular disease, primarily through controlling the level of the amino acid homocysteine in your blood. Preliminary research also shows folic acid may help protect against certain cancers and Alzheimer's. In March 2004, the Centers for Disease Control (CDC) released a paper reporting that, since folic acid fortification to enriched grains was mandated in 1998, there have been 31,000 fewer stroke-associated deaths and 17,000 fewer deaths related to ischemic heart disease in the United States each year.

HOW MUCH DO YOU NEED?

Your body cannot make folic acid, so it must be supplied in the diet. The Recommended Dietary Allowance (RDA) for folic acid is 400 micrograms (mcg.) per day. If women get 400 mcg. of folic acid in their diet before conception, their chances of having a baby born with a neural tube defect is greatly reduced. Since 1998, when the FDA implemented the policy that required fortification of enriched grain products with folic acid, the rate of neural tube defects has been reduced by 20 to 30 percent.

Folate found naturally in foods is not absorbed as well as folic acid from fortified foods or supplements. In addition to the naturally occurring folate you obtain from eating a varied diet, the Food and

Nutrition Board of the National Academy of Sciences recommends getting 400 micrograms of folic acid by:

+   Consuming foods fortified with folic acid (fortified breakfast cereals, fortified orange juice, and enriched grain foods such as bread, pasta, and rice)

+   Taking a multivitamin or supplement with folic acid

Since January 1, 1998, getting enough folic acid on a daily basis became a bit easier. By this date, the FDA required that all enriched grain foods be fortified with folic acid.

So do not despair if you think you might be falling short of folic acid. When you are having a bowl of cereal for breakfast or a sandwich made with white bread for lunch, or if you make a commitment to supplement your diet with a multivitamin containing folic acid, you will come closer to meeting the goal of 400 mcg. a day. And you can feel good about getting the folic acid you need in the foods you already enjoy.

THE FOLIC ACID FACTOR

If you are wondering how much folic acid you are getting from the foods you eat, take a look at the tables below.

Foods Fortified With Folic Acid		
Breads/Grains/Cereals	Serving Size	Folic Acid (mcg)
White bread, enriched	1 slice	34
Breakfast cereals, fortified	1 ounce	100–400*
Instant oatmeal	1 package	100
Pasta, enriched	½ cup	80

Rice, enriched	½ cup	60
Foods That Are Excellent Natural Sources of Folate**		
Fruits/Fruit Juice	Serving Size	Folate (mcg)
Orange juice	½ cup	37
Orange	1 medium	48
Strawberries	1 cup	80
Vegetables	Serving Size	Folate (mcg)
Spinach, cooked	½ cup	131
Spinach, raw	1 cup	29
Lentils, cooked	½ cup	179
Black/white beans, cooked	½ cup	125
Asparagus, cooked	6 spears	121
Meat/Poultry	Serving Size	Folate (mcg)
Chicken liver, simmered	¼ cup	269
Beef liver, cooked	3 oz.	184
Nuts	Serving Size	Folate (mcg)
Peanuts	1/3 cup	117
Sunflower seeds	1/2 cup	152

*Check the Nutrition Facts label to determine the exact amount of folic acid in the cereal you eat.

**The foods listed in this chart represent many of the best sources of folate. Folate is present in smaller amounts in other foods. Remember that folic acid is better absorbed than folate.

FAT

Despite the increasing popularity of low-carb (and relatively high-fat) diets, dietary fat still gets quite a bit of negative attention. After all, public health recommendations uniformly call for reducing intake of dietary fat. So it is easy to become fat-phobic and forget it is a nutrient necessary for good health. In moderate amounts, fat performs a variety of important functions in your body. It would not only be impossible—but also not good for your body—to live on a totally fat-free diet.

WHY DO YOU NEED FAT?

As described in Chapter 1, fat in your diet performs several important functions, including:

- Providing your body with energy (nine calories per gram).

- Helping your body absorb and transport certain vitamins (A, D, E, and K).

Fat in your diet may even help with appetite control—giving you a feeling of fullness and minimizing between-meal hunger pangs. However, evidence is clear that a diet high in fat, especially saturated and trans fat, relates to many chronic health problems; among them are heart disease, some types of cancer, diabetes, and obesity.

WHAT ARE THE DIFFERENT TYPES OF FAT?

SATURATED FAT

If you have a choice, saturated fats are the fats you want to consume less of. Numerous scientific reports link a high intake of saturated fat to higher blood cholesterol and a greater risk for heart disease.

Animal products such as meat, poultry, lard, and whole milk are the main sources of saturated fat, but you also can find them in palm and coconut oils. Foods high in saturated fatty acids are firm at room temperature.

TRANS FAT

Trans fat behaves like saturated fat in terms of its cholesterol-raising effects so, if you have a choice, you will want to consume less of this type of fat as well. Some researchers believe trans fats are even worse than saturated fat, because they—unlike saturated fats—tend to reduce HDL cholesterol (the good kind). Trans fat is a type of fat formed during the process of hydrogenation—when unsaturated oils are processed to make them stable and solid at room temperature. Recent methods have been developed to hydrogenate oils that are successful in not producing trans fats. Not all products that contain hydrogenated oils contain trans fats.

No official "safe" upper limit or recommendation has been established for trans fat. However, to give consumers more information when choosing foods, in July 2003, the FDA announced that food manufacturers will be required to list in the Nutrition Facts label the trans fat content of the product. This new FDA regulation officially starts January 1, 2006, and applies to packaged foods and also to some dietary supplements such as energy and nutrition bars.

In the meantime, some ways to reduce consumption of trans fats include:

- Choose margarines that come with a label indicating "zero trans fats."

- Use unhydrogenated oils rich in monounsaturated fats, such as canola and olive oil.

- Read ingredients on food labels. If you consume a lot of processed foods, watch for foods that have "hydrogenated vegetable oil" or "partially hydrogenated vegetable oil" as one of the first few ingredients listed as they may contain trans fats.

- Limit consumption of deep-fried foods such as french fries.

UNSATURATED FAT

Unsaturated fats are "better" fats, and they come in two forms. Both have been associated with a number of health benefits, including improved blood cholesterol.

- **Monounsaturated fatty acids (MUFA)**—Monounsaturated fats such as peanut oil, olive oil, and fish oils tend not to raise blood cholesterol levels and may even be beneficial in lowering them when used in place of saturated fats.

- **Polyunsaturated fatty acids (PUFA)**—Polyunsaturated fats such as safflower, sunflower, corn, soybean, sesame, and canola oils tend not to raise blood cholesterol.

- **Omega-3 fatty acids**—These fats are highly polyunsaturated. They are mostly found in seafood, especially higher-fat fish such as albacore tuna, mackerel, and salmon. Soybean and canola oil supply a different kind of omega-3s, too. Some research suggests that omega-3s may help prevent heart disease.

WHERE ARE UNSATURATED FATS FOUND?

You can find unsaturated fats in a variety of foods, including fish, nuts, olives, avocadoes, and oils. At room temperature, unsaturated fats are usually liquid.

All fats and oils actually contain a combination of all three major types of fat (saturated, monounsaturated, and polyunsaturated) in various proportions. The following chart shows these proportions. You will notice that canola, safflower, and sunflower oils are composed mainly of unsaturated fatty acids; whereas coconut oil, palm kernel oil, and butter contain primarily saturated fatty acids.

COMPARISON OF DIETARY FATS

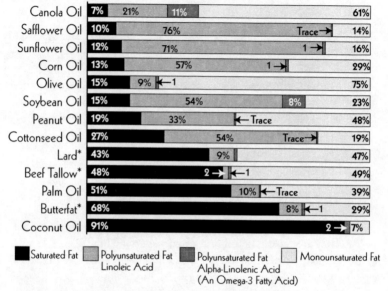

*Cholesterol content (mg/Tbsp): Lard 12; Beef tallow 14; Butterfat 33. No cholesterol in any vegetable-based oil.

Source: POS Pilot Plant Corporation, Saskatoon, Saskatchewan, Canada, June 1994

HOW MUCH FAT DO YOU NEED?

For most of us, the best approach is to eat a moderate amount of fat, primarily unsaturated fats. Many health organizations such as the American Dietetic Association, the American Heart Association, and the American Diabetes Association recommend aiming for:

- Less than 30 percent of total calories from fat.

- Less than 10 percent of total calories from saturated fat.

You are now more familiar with the nutrients your body needs for health and wellness! Here are a few tips from the Dietary Guidelines Alliance to help you expand your tastes, enjoy a variety of foods, and get the nutrients your body needs. Be adventurous!

- Go ahead—buy one fruit or vegetable you see at the grocery store that you have not tried before.

- Enjoy a meal at a Thai, Indian, Vietnamese, or Japanese restaurant.

- Prepare a new recipe from a favorite magazine or cookbook.

- Dig into a different grain such as couscous, bulgur, barley, or quinoa.

- Experiment with imaginative snacks, such as fruit kabobs with low-fat yogurt or air-popped popcorn lightly seasoned with herbs or Parmesan cheese.

CHAPTER FOUR

Recognizing and Maintaining Your Natural Weight

WHAT IS A NATURAL, COMFORTABLE, AND HEALTHY WEIGHT FOR YOU? THIS CHAPTER WILL ASSIST YOU IN ADOPTING BEHAVIORS THAT MAY HELP YOU BE SUCCESSFUL AT MANAGING YOUR WEIGHT.

IT IS AN INCREDIBLE contradiction: At the same time that super-thin, waif-like models have become the ideal, the number of Americans who are considered overweight (by the National Heart, Lung, and Blood Institute guidelines) has risen to more than half of the population.

Most of us—especially women—are conscious about our weight regardless of our current size or shape. Average body weights for fashion models, television and movie actresses, and beauty pageant contestants, have dropped during the past few decades. Because so few women can even come close to meeting today's cultural standard, weight obsession and "bad scale days" are more prevalent than ever before.

A thin body, however, is not necessarily best for everyone. In terms of health, one size does not fit all. Healthy bodies can come in many shapes and sizes. So what is your natural weight? It is essentially how much your body tends to weigh naturally, without dieting or excessive exercising. What constitutes a healthy, reasonable, and comfortable weight for you is not as simple as a number on a scale.

Many Americans are, undoubtedly, at a weight that is not best for them. Being truly over your natural, healthy weight is associated with a number of health risks. Through some easy measurements, you can get an indication of your risk for certain health problems, like heart disease and adult-onset diabetes.

DETERMINING YOUR WAIST MEASUREMENT

Where you carry your weight, and where you have gained the most weight over the years, is important to your health. Excess fat in your abdomen (intra-abdominal) is much more of a health risk than excess fat on your hips and thighs.

WHAT SHAPE ARE YOU?

Measure your waist while standing in a relaxed stance, without sucking in your abdomen. This measurement should reflect the largest circumference around your belly, which will typically be at the level of your navel. If you have a substantial amount of fat around your midsection, sometimes the navel tends to be located beneath that point. If your waist measurement exceeds the numbers below, it may indicate that you have an unhealthy amount of intra-abdominal fat, which may place you at high risk for heart disease and adult-onset diabetes.

HIGH-RISK WAIST MEASUREMENT

Men > 40 inches
Women > 35 inches

Source: "NHLBI Guidelines on the Identification, Evaluation, and Treatment of Overweight and Obesity in Adults," The Evidence Report, NIH Publication No. 98–4083.

BODY WEIGHT AND SET-POINT

Ideal weight for each person is unique, thanks to the unique genetic make-up of our body. One part of this uniqueness is set-point, the body weight within a range that each person tends to maintain over long periods of time, regardless of whether it is healthy or not. This helps explain why some people maintain a relatively stable weight without even trying, whereas millions of others keep returning to, more or less, the same weight despite perpetual efforts to change. Though we do not fully understand how set-point works, we do know that it operates with a fair amount of precision.

You may ask, "If the set-point really worked, why am I 10 pounds heavier than I was 10 years ago?" You are not alone. Because most adults in the United States do gain weight as they get older, this means that our set-point is flexible. It is best to think of your set-point not as a specific and rigid number, but the body weight within your set-point range that reflects your current lifestyle.

The closer you get to the limits of your set-point range, the more difficult it may be to maintain that weight. However, there is a lot you can do to determine where within the range you will be. Although genetics plays a role in determining your range, lifestyle—including physical activity and diet—significantly help determine where within that range you may be.

Sources: Harris, R.B., "Role of set-point theory in regulation of body weight." FASEB Journal, 4:3310-3318, 1990; Kessey, R.E., Powley, T.L., "The regulation of body weight" Ann. Rev. Psychol., 37:109–133, 1986.

SUCCESSFUL WEIGHT MANAGEMENT

Research has shown continually that the two most common features of maintaining a healthy weight are:

- Regular physical activity

Whether it is walking, climbing the stairs at work, hitting the gym, or joining a softball league, you have to move. Physically active persons are more able to maintain a healthful weight throughout life. Active persons are also less likely to regain pounds after weight loss.

- Maintaining a moderate intake of calories—following the recommendations of the Food Guide Pyramid

The key is to eat the amount of food your body needs to maintain a healthy weight. Eating according to the Food Guide Pyramid will naturally help you meet your goal of fewer than 30 percent of total daily calories from fat and consume the amount of calories you need.

ALSO—SET REALISTIC GOALS!

If you have set a goal to lose a certain number of pounds in two months and you are frustrated because you have not reached your goal, remember—it is possible that you are already at your natural weight. You may not need to lose more weight to achieve health benefits.

If you still want to lose weight, the best strategy is to make small changes over time in what you eat and in your level of activity. After all, small steps work better than giant leaps. Try setting a behavior goal rather than a weight goal. For example, make a goal of walking with a friend three times a week for 30 minutes. Or, start by choosing the stairs over the elevator at work. And focus on the process rather than the result!

IS WEIGHT LOSS REALLY NECESSARY?

Before making a decision about losing weight, ask yourself the following questions. Mark each question with "yes" or "no," and then select the scenario that best represents your answers. Be honest with yourself.

1. Do I get at least 30 minutes of moderate-intensity activity on most days of the week? In other words, am I physically active enough to achieve health benefits? (See Chapter 6) Yes _____ No _____

2. Do I follow the recommendations of the Food Guide Pyramid?
    Yes _____ No _____

3. Do I have any medical conditions that are weight-related (e.g.,
    high blood pressure, elevated triglycerides, glucose intolerance,
    adult-onset diabetes, osteoarthritis)?   Yes _____ No _____

4. Since the age of 20, has my body weight increased by more than
    about five pounds per decade (i.e., about one-half pound per
    year)?   Yes _____ No _____

INTERPRETING YOUR ANSWERS

Find the scenario below that most closely represents your answers.

SCENARIO 1

YES to questions 1 and 2 NO to questions 3 and 4

If your weight has remained reasonably stable ± 5 pounds of your
adult weight) throughout your adult life, you are active, and you eat
a balanced, varied diet, your current weight is probably a healthful
weight for you. If you are active, eat nutritiously, and have no weight-
related medical problems, your natural, biologically preferred weight
may (or may not) be heavier than the normal range for the population. Remember—normal for the population may not be right for
you. There are no compelling health or medical reasons to try to lose
weight.

If you are not content with your weight, you may want to evaluate
why. If your weight is within the normal range for your height, and
you would still like to be slimmer than you are now, try:

•   Gradually increasing your physical activity level.

•   Focusing your energy on body acceptance rather than losing
    weight.

• Making some changes in your diet to help you achieve a healthful weight loss.

Scenario 2
YES to all questions

You should consult your physician regardless of your current weight (or whether you are content with your current weight). Having a medical condition, like high blood pressure, needs professional treatment. Your current level of physical activity, and/or the extent to which you follow the Food Guide Pyramid, also may not be sufficient for optimal health. For some men and women, higher levels of physical activity and/or more aggressive dietary strategies may be necessary to correct medical problems. You may decide to consult a registered dietitian or certified fitness professional for help with your diet and physical activity.

Scenario 3
YES to questions 1, 2, and 4 NO to question 3

The weight you have gained during your adult life is most likely not unhealthy. It could reflect periods of your life when you were more sedentary and/or had eating habits that were conducive to gaining weight. It also may reflect weight gained during pregnancy that was not all lost after childbirth. If you have decided to lose weight for a reason other than health, gradually:

• Increase your physical activity level (i.e., go for an after-dinner walk with your children).

• Make some changes in your diet to help you achieve a healthful weight loss (i.e., enjoying a piece of fruit or half a bagel instead of chips for a snack).

Scenario 4
NO to either question 1 or 2 NO to questions 3 and 4

A sedentary lifestyle—the norm for most of us office workers—and a poor diet are significant risk factors for future health problems and premature death, regardless of weight. Even though you have gained little, if any, weight since the age of 20, you are not immune to health problems. Regardless of your answers to questions 3 and 4, your health and overall well-being may be even better if you become more active and follow the recommendations of the Food Guide Pyramid.

SCENARIO 5

NO to either question 1 or 2 YES to either question 3 or 4

Your current weight may not be the most healthful weight for you (but it could be!). It is difficult to tell if you are at your natural weight if you are not taking good care of yourself. If your weight is outside the normal range for your height, and you have health problems frequently associated with excess weight, then you probably are over your natural weight. A combination of being overweight and either a sedentary lifestyle or an unbalanced diet significantly increases your health risks. However, even if you are within the normal range on standard height/weight tables, you may not necessarily be healthy. Although a return to the body weight you had at age 20 is improbable, becoming more physically active and following the dietary recommendations of the Food Guide Pyramid, can greatly improve your health, as well as help you achieve and maintain a healthful weight.

WEIGHT-LOSS READINESS TEST

There are behaviors that need to be in place for anyone who has struggled with food or weight before a change can ever happen. Place a check mark next to the behaviors that you practice on a consistent basis. Be honest with yourself. The answers should reflect the way you really think—not how you would like to be.

☐   I understand why I might be eating more than my body needs.

☐ I know how to keep a food journal (see Chapter 4) to record food, my feelings, and hunger/satiety.

☐ I usually keep a food journal when I am having a hard time with my food/weight.

☐ I am in tune with my hunger and am comfortable beginning most of my meals hungry.

☐ I am able to stop eating when physically satisfied, usually with no problem.

☐ I am able to eat almost any food without beating myself up or feeling guilty.

I almost always take action to handle feelings and situations that trigger me to eat by ...

☐ identifying the feeling/situation.

☐ making a choice between feeling uncomfortable or addressing the issue.

☐ making effective changes on my own, when possible.

☐ reaching out for appropriate support from family and friends.

☐ engaging in counseling if I see my reaction to triggers not changing.

☐ My attitude toward my body is "if you can't be with the one you love, love the one you're with."

☐   I practice nurturing behaviors (self-care) to satisfy myself so that I do not need to turn to food.

☐   I usually know what my needs are and how to get them met by setting limits and communicating directly.

☐   I usually assert myself and rarely have to resort to yelling, arguing, or withdrawing when feeling frustrated with others around me.

☐   I like my body most of the time.

☐   I realize when "I feel fat," an issue other than weight needs to be addressed.

☐   I know that if I lose weight to feel better, that "feeling better" is almost always transient since it is not the weight loss that makes me feel better, but what I think about the weight loss. I can feel better right now by changing the way I think.

☐   I have changed the way I think and feel content with myself most of the time.

If you are consistently practicing the behaviors above, you may be ready to make a change. Remember, going on a "diet" is the quickest prescription for eventual weight gain for most people.

Source: Karin Kratina, M.A., R.D., adapted from the unpublished work of Peggy DeMars M.S.,R.D.

CHAPTER FIVE

How Much Do I Need To Eat?

Is it possible to moderate your own food intake and maintain a natural weight? This chapter shows you how to regulate your food intake, enjoy food and eating, and still maintain your weight and sanity. And, yes, this includes eating carbs, too! After all, in terms of weight, it's the calories, not the carbs, that count.

It is ironic how basic needs, like eating, can become more distorted the older we get. As infants and young children, we are naturally attuned to our body's signals of hunger and fullness, what we call "natural eating." Later in life, as we begin to diet or control our food intake, our eating habits become anything but natural. We start to diet, gain weight, diet more in response, and find ourselves involved in a vicious cycle—one that all too often results in eating less and less, binging in response, weighing more and more, and gradually losing any sense of pleasure or natural control in relation to food. Diets teach people to focus on what they eat, rather than how they eat, yet it is our relationship with food that most determines if we are eating more than our body is asking for.

Diets also tend to divide foods into "good" and "bad," with avoidance of the so-called "bad" foods being the key to weight loss. This is certainly true of the low-carb diets so popular today, which ask dieters to shun foods that make up approximately one-half the calories they typically consume (and rely on for proper nutrients). But it is not necessary to eliminate entire food groups to maintain a healthy body weight. All foods can fit into a healthy diet.

Many typical nutrition books look at food strictly in terms of calories and nutrients. This is just fine if you view the body as a simple input-output machine. From the standpoint of weight control, calories *do* count; calorie counting, however, is a very tedious task, and one that few can stay with for any length of time. Although calories do count, you do not have to count them. And the elimination of entire food groups has never proven successful in the long term (as the first go-around with low-carb dieting a few decades ago demonstrated).

We want to increase your awareness of other "issues" that exist when you eat. For example, eating styles can be divided into four categories: Attuned Eating, Misguided Eating, Deprivation-Driven Eating, and Emotional Eating. The following quiz is designed to help you better understand how people can have different relationships with food and to help you see more clearly what your relationship with food might be.

WORKSHEET: NUTRITION BEYOND THE FOOD GUIDE PYRAMID—DIFFERENT EATING STYLES

Check the following statements that are true for you:	Usually True	Sometimes True	Almost Never True
Style One:			
I eat only when I am hungry.	——	——	——
It is clear to me when I am hungry, although sometimes it is so automatic, I don't even think about it.	——	——	——
I know when to quit eating because I feel satisfied.	——	——	——

	Usually True	Sometimes True	Almost Never True

I usually stop eating because I seem to lose interest in food as I get full.

Sometimes I eat until I am full, sometimes I eat until I am satisfied, but I am clear on what the difference is.

Style Two:

I really don't pay attention to when I am hungry.

I quit eating when the plate is "clean."

I often eat "just because it is there."

I often realize I am hungry when food is put in front of me.

I really don't pay much attention to feeling full.

Style Three:

I feel deprived of foods, and may eat just because those foods are available.

I try to restrict my food intake because I do not want to overeat.

I get so hungry that all food looks good.

I stop eating because I tell myself that I should.

	Usually True	Sometimes True	Almost Never True
I frequently eat until I feel "overfull," even though I have every intention of stopping much earlier.	___	___	___
I eat more now because I know I will not let myself have any later.	___	___	___
Style Four:			
It is hard for me to tell when I am physically hungry.	___	___	___
I feel "hungry" very soon after eating what most people would consider a decent meal.	___	___	___
I don't like to stop eating, even if I am full.	___	___	___
I eat until I am numb.	___	___	___
I eat when I am upset.	___	___	___

SCORING

Give yourself:
2 points for every "Usually True"
1 point for every "Sometimes True"
0 points for every "Almost Never True"

Add up your points and record them below:
Style One: _____

Style Two: _____
Style Three: _____
Style Four: _____

- If you scored highest for Style One and scored very low on all other styles, you are an **Attuned Eater.**

- If you scored highest for Style Two, you are a **Misguided Eater.**

- If you scored highest for Style Three, you are a **Deprivation-Driven Eater.**

- If you scored highest for Style Four, you are an **Emotional Eater.**

Source: Karin Kratina, M.A., R.D., Renfrew Center of South Florida, adapted from work of Ellyn Satter, M.S., R.D.

STYLES OF EATING

While most people are a mixture of several eating styles, you may find you tend more toward one style than the others.

STYLES OF EATING: ATTUNED EATER

If you are an Attuned Eater, lucky you! You are one of the "normal eaters" who eats in response to physical hunger. As you eat, you gradually experience a sense of satisfaction. This is your body telling you the hunger is gone. You are probably at your natural weight and do not worry much about losing or maintaining your weight. You usually eat when you are hungry and stop eating when satisfied, seldom eating when you are not hungry. You rarely eat emotionally, but when you do, you do not usually eat again until you are hungry. You never deprive yourself of specific foods, but you do consider nutrition when choosing your foods.

Attuned Eaters often have fairly healthy diets, but can occasionally benefit from "fine-tuning" the diet. Since you have little emotional investment in food, it is usually easy to make any recommended improvements in your diet.

Tips For Optimizing Nutrition: Attuned Eater

Compare what you eat to the Food Guide Pyramid

To fine tune your diet, compare the food and beverages you consume over the course of a day to the Food Guide Pyramid. The food diary at the end of this chapter will make this more convenient. You may want to copy it and keep track for several days to get a better idea of what you are eating. Aim to make any adjustments necessary to be sure you are getting the minimum recommendations.

Styles of Eating: Misguided Eater

If you are a Misguided Eater, you probably have not dieted a great deal, although you may have reduced your food intake on occasion to drop some weight. You sometimes eat emotionally, but not often. You are concerned about your nutritional intake, but have a great deal of misinformation.

Misguided Eaters are able to use internal cues of hunger and satiety to determine when and how much to eat, but tend to ignore these signals or not notice them. As a result, they easily eat when not hungry, especially if food happens to be available. As a Misguided Eater, you may not be aware of hunger until you see food, when you suddenly realize that you are indeed quite hungry. It is not unusual for you to continue eating beyond the point of satisfaction. The classic Misguided Eater is a charter member of the Clean Plate Club.

The flip side of the Clean Plate Club is the Pre-Packaged Portion Club, filled with Misguided Eaters who stop eating because the pre-portioned meal (a low-calorie frozen meal, for instance) is supposed to be enough to satisfy. When hunger returns too soon before the next meal, these Misguided Eaters may conclude that something is wrong with them or their will power.

The Misguided Eater often finds it difficult to access and discuss feelings, especially uncomfortable feelings, and tends not to pay attention to hunger and satiety. Although looking at deeper feelings would benefit Misguided Eaters, they are often able to improve nutritional intake with basic nutrition information and increased awareness of hunger and satiety cues.

Tips for Optimizing Nutrition: Misguided Eater

Practice "Attuned Eating"

Eat when you are physically hungry and stop when you are satisfied most of the time. Slow down and tune in to your body's signals.

Use the Food Guide Pyramid to challenge your beliefs about food and ensure you are getting enough

Compare what you eat to the Food Guide Pyramid recommendations to ensure your diet is healthy. Try to eat a wide variety of foods and be sure you have plenty of delicious, healthy food available to you.

STYLES OF EATING: DEPRIVATION-DRIVEN EATER

As a Deprivation-Driven Eater, you may have been on restrictive nutritional or weight-loss regimens and react to that deprivation by feeling out of control around food or thoughts of food. You may have been encouraged to divide foods into "good" and "bad" (or "legal" and "illegal") foods and have tried very hard to be a "good" ("legal") eater. As a result, you find it very difficult to hear your internal cues of hunger and satiety and, therefore, need an external structure to help you decide when and how much to eat. All this manipulation of food and eating robs you of the opportunity to:

- Be relaxed around food

- Respond to the body's cues of hunger and satiety in a natural way

- Walk away from food simply because you are satisfied (not full, but satisfied) and just do not want anymore

Deprivation-Driven Eaters may be fearful that they will not stay full after a meal, making it difficult for them to stop eating when satisfied. Deprivation-Driven Eaters often have idealistic notions about the "right" way to eat. Interestingly, they often fall short of a healthy food plan because they do not allow for sufficient food. As a Deprivation-Driven Eater, you need to let go of the "diet mentality" and begin to eat in a way that nourishes both your body and your awareness of it. The tools of deprivation with which you are familiar—identifying healthy options, counting calories or fat grams, or developing an individualized food plan—will most likely be counterproductive for you.

TIPS FOR OPTIMIZING NUTRITION: DEPRIVATION-DRIVEN EATER

Stop dieting right away

Not only can you manage your weight without dieting, you can actually manage your weight more effectively if you are not dieting. Simply dealing with Deprivation-Driven Eating and Emotional Eating is sometimes enough to establish your natural weight.

Move away from a diet mentality

- Stop buying "diet" foods. Diet foods promote a "diet mentality" of counting calories or fat, weighing on scales, and generally obsessing about body size. These concerns do not promote health.

- Throw out the scale. Many people use the scale to determine how "good" or "bad" they have been. Like calorie counting, the all-powerful scale can get in the way of the relaxed attitude that contributes to healthy eating.

- Legalize all food. When you have treats, enjoy them. "Forbidden" foods are the ones that haunt you—the first things you look for on a menu. It is only natural for you to want these foods even more than you would if they had not been restricted. By not avoiding any food, you can spend more time thinking about what you do want to have—whether it is food or something else entirely.

Practice "Attuned Eating"

Eat when you are physically hungry and stop when you are satisfied most of the time. Do not allow yourself to get too hungry since it is easier to stop eating if you do not start out extremely hungry. It may help to carry food you enjoy with you so you do not have to be concerned about becoming too hungry.

STYLES OF EATING: EMOTIONAL EATER

If you are an Emotional Eater, you separate food from hunger to satisfy certain emotional needs. You respond to emotions by either overeating or undereating, your weight fluctuating as a result. There may be times when you never feel full because you instead "go unconscious," numbing the physical pain or discomfort that signal the very extremes of fullness.

Emotional Eaters may or may not be in touch with their signals of hunger and satiety, but they often find themselves eating without considering these cues. This type of eating is an important coping mechanism in which people reach for food outside the bounds of hunger and satiety as a way of gaining a sense of security, freedom from anxiety, or relief from feelings that seem out of control (such as anger, sadness, or happiness). It may include eating beyond satisfaction, through fullness, and into pain.

Emotional "Undereaters" are seldom in touch with their hunger and will comment that they just never feel hungry. Actually, they are numbing out and staying as far away from feelings as possible.

Because it is impossible to selectively ignore certain feelings and sensations while staying in touch with others, numbing out in one area means that feelings in all areas are numb, including the areas of hunger and satiety.

Tips for Optimizing Nutrition: Emotional Eater

Move away from a diet mentality (see description under Deprivation-Driven Eater above)

Use a food journal with a hunger scale

Use the Hunger/Satiety Scale and Food Journal at the end of this chapter to help you differentiate between emotional "hunger" and physical hunger.

Your stomach is like a gas tank

- "0" is empty, no fuel. The car has nothing to go on. You are ravenous, maybe even a bit faint with hunger.

- "10" is filled to the brim. You could not possibly add another drop of gas—"Thanksgiving full."

- "5" is a neutral place, neither so empty that you are worried about running out of gas, nor so full that you feel you could drive forever.

- At "4," you are a little hungry.

- At "6," there is no hunger, but if you quit eating now, you will be hungry again in a couple of hours.

Take a moment to relax, close your eyes, and focus on the sensations in your stomach. Where on the scale are you right now?

Hunger and satiety are subjective. One person may describe a "3" as dizzy and lightheaded; another may describe it as a strong desire for food.

Practice "Attuned Eating"

Eat when you are physically hungry and stop when you are satisfied most of the time. Sometimes it is difficult for Emotional Overeaters to experience hunger because, when they get to a "4" on the hunger scale, they start getting nervous—a conditioned response to the fear of hunger. If you find that you need to eat at a "4" or "5," be very gentle with yourself. Practice just once a day going to a "3." Have your next meal planned so that the "3" does not feel too out of control.

Do not allow yourself to get too hungry; it is easier to stop eating if you do not start out extremely hungry. You might want to carry food you enjoy with you so you are not preoccupied with becoming too hungry.

Emotional "Undereaters" are often able to reconnect with hunger and satiety if they eat sufficient food for a week or two. This may mean sometimes eating when you do not feel like it.

Decode non-physical "hunger"

Being aware of hunger and satiety cues, then eating in response to them, makes it so much easier to find out why you want to eat when you are not really hungry. When you are physically at a "7," yet feel extremely hungry, your feeling of hunger is communicating something. You are not really physically hungry, so what exactly are you hungry for? What are you communicating about yourself?

For many of us, eating is often a way of controlling or containing our feelings; Emotional Eaters, for example, frequently use food to act out their emotions. By "decoding" this emotional eating, you can learn a great deal about what is going on in your life that drives your nonphysical hunger. Although your hunger is complex and unique, certain broad patterns can be identified in the meaning of your non-physical hunger.

Once you have figured out why you want to eat when you are not really hungry, you may be tempted to decide simply to stop emotional eating. However, this can be counterproductive because the need you were expressing through the hunger is left unaddressed. Instead, the next time you are at a "7" and want to eat, remember, for example, this hunger, in the past, meant you were angry with your husband and afraid to tell him. You might choose to eat cheesecake and not confront your husband, or you might choose to sit down and resolve your anger, either face to face with your husband or by talking it over with a friend. Decoding gives you the power to choose.

It is normal for people to eat for enjoyment, entertainment, and even out of anger on occasion. But when food becomes a primary means of coping with unmet needs, decoding can help restore the missing balance.

Ensure adequate intake, using the Food Guide Pyramid

When you are caught up in emotional eating, it is very difficult to eat healthfully. It is very important to get at least the minimum recommendations from the Food Guide Pyramid whenever possible. Be sure you are getting ENOUGH food so you are not overly hungry. (If you find it difficult to take in enough food, follow the guidelines for **Ensuring adequate intake, using the Food Guide Pyramid for the Deprivation-Driven Eater.**)

Work with a registered dietitian and therapist

If you find it difficult to differentiate between emotional eating and your physical needs; if you are unable to get in touch with hunger and satiety; or, if you are unsure of how to utilize the Food Guide Pyramid, it may be helpful to meet with a registered dietitian. Make sure he or she is skilled at working with hunger and satiety and differentiating between emotional and physical hunger, and make sure your treatment will not consist simply of a structured meal plan to follow. Sometimes, working with a skilled psychotherapist can help you pinpoint your emotional needs and determine how to meet them without food. Be sure the therapist has some experience working with emotional eating issues.

PRACTICE SUPPORTIVE EATING

Throw out the terms "good" and "bad." All too often, we feel bad about eating potato chips, but feel we have been good if we order a plain baked potato. These words stigmatize food choices in ways that are destructive of natural, attuned eating. Take a look at these two situations.

A mother is chatting with her child in the evening, just before bedtime. They have both eaten the minimums from the Food Guide Pyramid and both had dessert after dinner. While they talk, they each have a couple of chocolate kisses. Is the chocolate good or bad?

What about this situation? The mother, who enjoys chocolate, views it as "fattening," so she has carrot sticks instead. As she talks with her child, she feels deprived and does not enjoy the carrots. Faced with her child's obvious enjoyment of the chocolate, she has a hard time focusing on the conversation they are sharing. Are the carrots good or bad?

In this scenario, chocolate can be a positive way for a mother and child to bond through a shared pleasure. Carrots can't substitute for the pleasure of chocolate. In fact, the mother's preoccupation with the carrots is distracting her, so she is not enjoying the time spent with her child. Health includes emotions, relationships, and a sense of connectedness, just as much as it does good nutrition.

Instead of the terms "good" and "bad," try using "supportive" and "non-supportive." Ask yourself, "Would eating this food be supportive (or not supportive) for me at this time?" The answer may not always be clear-cut, but that is all right. It is not always easy to abandon assumptions that cake is bad, while broccoli is good. Here is how you might answer the question, "Would a piece of cake be supportive for me?" on various occasions:

- "Well, no, not really. I am having a hard time getting enough protein today. I will have a serving from the milk group then see if I am still hungry for cake. If not, I can always have it tomorrow."

- "Yes, I think it would. I will be able to get in the rest of the food groups I need at dinner. I am at a '6' on the hunger scale now, so if I don't have the cake, I will be hungry in the middle of work. A piece of cake sounds good right now."

- "Gee, I am really frustrated and angry. The cake would calm me down—for a minute. Then I will just need more cake. I think I will take a stroll before going back to work; maybe that will take care of some of this anger."

- "Gosh, I feel really stressed out. I am not sure cake is the most supportive thing I could do right now. But I know I am going to eat it anyway, so I will make this as supportive as possible: I will get a glass of milk, turn off the TV, sit down at the dinner table with a nice napkin, and really enjoy this cake. Then I will take a minute to check in with myself and see if that was what I really wanted. If it wasn't, I will use that information next time!"

HINTS FOR CREATING AN ENJOYABLE EATING EXPERIENCE

Enjoyable eating and healthful eating go hand in hand. Enjoyable eating primarily stems from being free to explore and experiment with food, recognizing the sensual aspects of the food experience. Healthful eating primarily stems from identifying, interpreting, and meeting physical needs. Those who are able to be attuned to their eating report more healthful diets, as well as more pleasant eating experiences.

TRY THE FOLLOWING SUGGESTIONS:

- **When you eat, savor the flavor and focus on enjoying the food.** If you find you are not enjoying it, ask yourself why you are eating it. If you find you are trying to eat more healthful foods but you do not like some of them, remember that sometimes it takes eating a food several different times to make it more familiar and, thus, more tasty.

- **Focus on the food.** Try not to do anything else while you are eating. When was the last time you sat down to a meal or snack and just ate—no book, no TV, no crossword puzzle, no radio—just focused on the tastes and smells of the food? While we pride ourselves on multi-tasking, doing this with our meals means we lose out on the pleasure of eating and we feel unsatisfied when finished eating. Before you eat, notice how it feels to be hungry. Focus on the food as you eat, pay attention to the taste and texture and your sense of being filled by the food. Notice how the hunger is gradually satisfied and how your body signals it has had enough to eat.

- **In between meals, notice how hunger returns.** Trust that you will be able to eat again in a way that will satisfy you and your hunger.

- **Focus on the present moment and appreciate the eating experience.** Try putting your fork down after each bite, consciously chewing, tasting, and swallowing each bite before taking the next. Your meals become more enjoyable, it becomes easier to listen to the body as hunger leaves, and it becomes easier to stop eating when you are satisfied.

- **Listen to your body's signals.** Notice how good food tastes when you are hungry. Notice how pleasure decreases as you get full.

- **Make eating special.** Treat yourself as you would an honored guest. This may mean setting an attractive table with candles and your best china and silverware. Arrange the food attractively on your plate, adding a garnish. Or it may mean you buy the best of the best … the best ice cream, the best strawberries. Savor each bite.

- **Remember, cheesecake can't make you fat.** But if you repeatedly eat cheesecake without considering hunger and satiety cues from your body, then you may gain weight.

MAKING "ATTUNED EATING" WORK FOR YOU

You may find yourself resisting attuned eating at first, especially if you have dieted a great deal or had lifelong food issues, but with practice, it becomes more and more rewarding. You will notice you are focusing on food less and, in all likelihood, eating less and enjoying it more. Along with this comes the most incredible freedom … a healthy life free of food issues.

USING A HUNGER/SATIETY RATING SCALE

Directions: Rate your hunger level before you eat and again when you are finished eating. It could look like a graph.* If you do this each time you eat, you will become more familiar with your eating patterns, especially if you discuss it with another person. Move away from using your head to decide your eating patterns and move toward listening to your body.

BASIC HUNGER/SATIETY SCALE

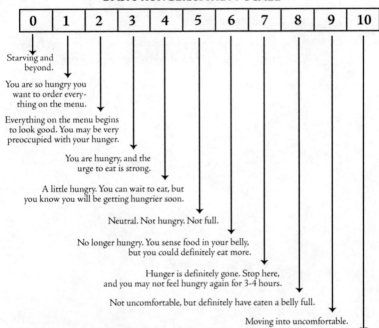

| 0 | 1 | 2 | 3 | 4 | 5 | 6 | 7 | 8 | 9 | 10 |

Starving and
beyond.

You are so hungry you
want to order every-
thing on the menu.

Everything on the menu begins
to look good. You may be very
preoccupied with your hunger.

You are hungry, and the
urge to eat is strong.

A little hungry. You can wait to eat, but
you know you will be getting hungrier soon.

Neutral. Not hungry. Not full.

No longer hungry. You sense food in your belly,
but you could definitely eat more.

Hunger is definitely gone. Stop here,
and you may not feel hungry again for 3-4 hours.

Not uncomfortable, but definitely have eaten a belly full.

Moving into uncomfortable.

Use description loosely and feel free to refine them with your counselor.

"Thanksgiving full". Very uncomfortable, maybe even painful.

Example:

0	1	2	3	4	5	6	7	8	9	10
			■	■	■	■	■			
						■	■	■		
		■	■	■	■	■	■	■	■	

The graphs represent:

A meal where you eat from 3-7.

A meal where you begin eating when you were not hungry, eating from 6-8

Eating from 2-9, from very hungry to uncomfortably full.

Source: Karin Kratina, M.A., R.D.

USING A FOOD JOURNAL WITH A HUNGER SCALE

Create a food journal to focus on your body's sensations of hunger, satisfaction, and fullness. The samples already filled in on the following pages will help give you an idea of how to complete your own.

FOOD JOURNAL—sample A

NAME: _Elinor_
DATE: _11 - 2 - 99_
DAY: M T W Th F Sa Su

FOOD JOURNAL

Today's Goal and/or Affirmation: _Eat when hungry, quit when satisfied._

TIME	FOOD AND QUANTITY	DP	B/MP	F/V	G	O	HUNGER SCALE	MOOD THOUGHTS AND/OR FEELINGS
8 am	1 cup cereal 1 cup skim milk 1 glass orange juice	1		1	2			This filled me up. Was really paying attention and feel satisfied.
11:00	1 apple and 6 crackers			1	2			Not very hungry, but lunch is late. Feeling rushed, ate this on the run.
1:30	1 bean burrito (large)		1	1	2			
2:00	2 mint candies					2		Just wanted something sweet. This is not emotional, even though I'm eating when not hungry.
6:00	4" sq piece of lasagna (w/veg) 2 cup salad with IT dressing 1 dinner roll cantaloupe 4 cookies	1	1	1 2 1	1 1	 4		Good dinner! Cantaloupe sweet. Still feeling rushed. Brought work home. Ugh! 8:00 Thinking about food, but I'm not a "7" so I know I'm not hungry.
9:30	1 pc of cake and glass of milk	1				1		Not at all hungry. Definately emotional, I know I won't gain weight if I wait until I'm hungry to eat again, so that's okay. I just need to deal with this stress!!!
TOTALS		3	2	7	8	7		
RECOMMENDED		2	2	6	9	7		EXERCISE: Hey, I didn't exercise, maybe a walk would help my stress!

DP = Dairy Products
B/MP = Bean/Meat Protein
F/V = Fruit/Vegetable
G = Grain
O = Others

HUNGER SCALE
0 1 2 3 4 5 6 7 8 9 10
0 = Empty
5 = Neutral
10 = Stuffed
Graph hunger level from start to end of meal.

FOOD JOURNAL—SAMPLE B

NAME: _Dana_
DATE: _8 - 10 - 99_
DAY: M T W Th F Sa Su

FOOD JOURNAL

Today's Goal and/or Affirmation:
Drop some weight!!

DP = Dairy Products
B/MP = Bean/Meat Protein
F/V = Fruit/Vegetable
G = Grain
O = Others

Hunger scale:
0 = Empty
5 = Neutral
10 = Stuffed
Graph hunger level from start to end of meal.

TIME	FOOD AND QUANTITY	DP	B/MP	F/V	G	O	HUNGER SCALE	MOOD, THOUGHTS AND/OR FEELINGS
8:00	1 cup cereal 1 cup milk	1			2			Really committed to dropping these 10 pounds.
10:00	1 apple			1				Gees, am really hungry, but doing good.
12:00	1 turkey sandwich		1	1	2			Doing good!!! Stayed below a "6." I'm really in control, feeling good.
3:00	3 granola bars				3	1		Why does it always happen that when I get real hungry I always overeat? I just need to diet better. No dinner for you!! Ate too much already.
	2 bagels				4			
10:30	2 bowls ice cream 12 graham crackers 6 peanut butter crackers				2	2		I was so hungry. Gees, I'm so weak willed. Why can't I stay on my diet.
TOTALS		1	1	2	13	3		**EXERCISE:**
RECOMMENDED		2	2	7	9			

CHAPTER SIX

The Importance of Physical Activity and Fitness in Health

How much exercise do you need? How intense should your workouts be? How can you fit physical activity into your schedule? This chapter will answer these questions and help you move toward your goal of becoming fit and healthy.

> "Eating alone will not keep a woman well; she must also take exercise. For food and exercise, while possessing opposite qualities, yet, work together to produce good health."
> Hippocrates, circa 400 B.C.

The wisdom of Hippocrates has become very apparent as we enter the new century. Countless studies from around the world show that being physically active on a regular basis significantly reduces the risk of many of our most prevalent diseases and also greatly enhances the quality of our lives. Exercise has been shown to have many health benefits—lowering blood pressure and cholesterol, and helping to decrease the risk of diseases like diabetes and osteoporosis. There also is evidence that exercise improves mood and psychological well-being and enhances self-esteem, while at the same time decreases stress, anxiety, and depression.

HOW MUCH PHYSICAL ACTIVITY IS ENOUGH?

To improve the health of Americans, the National Academy of Sciences now recommends the following:

"To maintain cardiovascular health at a maximal level, regardless of weight, adults and children ... should spend a total of at least one hour each day in moderately intense physical activity."

What does it mean to be physically active? How intense is moderate? And what does it mean to be fit? Research has shown quite conclusively that physical activity and fitness both are important determinants of our overall health and well-being.

- **Physical activity** refers to the very act of doing something—any voluntary body movement that burns calories, whether slowly over a long period of time, or fast and furious in just a few minutes. The intensity of the effort is how much it elevates your metabolism (i.e., calories per minute) and heart rate; whereas,

- **Physical fitness** refers to a more specific set of criteria and is defined most frequently in terms of aerobic fitness, muscular fitness, and flexibility.

Quite literally, you can take steps to become more physically active. To more fully appreciate the roles of physical activity and physical fitness in health, take a look at the chart below.

THE PHYSICAL ACTIVITY FITNESS CONTINUUM

HOW IT RELATES TO HEALTH AND FITNESS

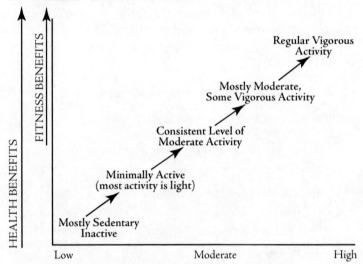

You will see that *any activity is better than no activity.*

- The health benefits of becoming more active begin almost right away by becoming at least "minimally active" (see left side of chart above). So, every little bit helps!

- The biggest health benefits are seen when you move to a level of consistent, moderate-intensity physical activity.

- Fitness benefits—and further health benefits—are observed when you move into the range of vigorous activity.

PHYSICAL ACTIVITY LEVEL

Mostly Sedentary/Inactive:

Health risk is very high. In fact, the American Heart Association now recognizes sedentary lifestyle as a risk factor for heart disease that is equal to the impact of smoking, high blood pressure, or elevated cholesterol.

- Your leisure-time activities involve little movement.

- You do not engage in sports or active recreational activities.

- You do not engage in any regular physical activity or exercise program of any kind.

- Your typical 24-hour day involves eating, sleeping, working at a sedentary job, watching TV, little, if any, walking, and relying almost exclusively on the automobile for transportation.

Minimally Active:

Health risk is still fairly high; active enough to achieve some health benefits.

- What little activity you engage in is mostly light (i.e., a stroll-pace walk once or twice per week).

- You do not engage in sports (except for the occasional July 4th softball game).

- Your typical 24-hour day is much like that of a sedentary person.

Consistent Level of Moderate Activity:

Active enough to achieve significant health benefits.

- You accumulate 30 minutes of moderate activity most days of the week.

- You do not engage in any structured exercise program, but make an effort to build physical activity into your day (i.e., fitting in short walks—even if only a few minutes—in your daily routine).

Mostly Moderate, Some Vigorous Activity:

Active enough to achieve significant health and fitness benefits.

- You often exercise beyond 30 minutes of moderate activity.

- You engage in aerobic activities.

- You occasionally engage in vigorous sports activities.

- You may include strength exercises as part of your physical activity

Regular Vigorous Activity:

Active enough to achieve significant health and fitness benefits.

- You may find vigorous activity challenging and rewarding.

- You routinely make aerobic and strength-building exercises part of your physical activity.

- You also may engage in vigorous sports activities.

The U.S. Department of Health and Human Services (DHHS) has found that the majority of U.S. adults fall into the first two categories, either completely sedentary or minimally active. Also, an estimated 70 to 80 percent of U.S. adults are not active enough to achieve health benefits.

WHAT IS THE DIFFERENCE BETWEEN "LIGHT," "MODERATE," AND "VIGOROUS" ACTIVITY?

- **Light** activities require less than 200 calories per hour and might be expected to increase your heart rate by less than 10 to 20 beats per minute.

- **Moderate** activities will burn between 200 to 400 calories per hour for most people and generally will increase your heart rate by no more than 20 to 40 beats per minute.

- **Vigorous** activities generally will burn more than 400 calories per hour and will, in most instances, increase your heart rate to >60 percent of maximum capacity.

QUIZ: HOW DOES MY ACTIVITY RATE?

Check the activities in which you participate on a daily/almost daily basis.

Light	Moderate	Vigorous
❑ Eating	❑ Bicycling, <10 mph	❑ Bicycling, >10 mph
❑ Washing dishes	❑ Line dancing, folk dancing, ballroom dancing	❑ Jogging, running
❑ Cooking	❑ Water aerobics	❑ Racquet sports
❑ Shopping	❑ Brisk walking, 3–4 mph	❑ Aerobic dancing
❑ Ironing	❑ Fishing and hunting	❑ Swimming
❑ Grooming, while sitting or standing	❑ Home repair, most activities	❑ Brisk walking, uphill with a load

- ❏ Talking on phone, standing
- ❏ Gardening, most activities
- ❏ Backpacking
- ❏ Playing most musical instruments
- ❏ Table tennis
- ❏ Rope skipping
- ❏ Slow walking, 1–2 mph
- ❏ Softball
- ❏ Roller blading or skating
- ❏ Playing darts
- ❏ Basketball, shooting baskets
- ❏ Touch football
- ❏ Bowling
- ❏ Frisbee
- ❏ Basketball, game
- ❏ Fishing (sitting)
- ❏ Horseback riding
- ❏ Skiing, downhill or cross-country
- ❏ Watering lawn
- ❏ Volleyball
- ❏ Shoveling snow
- ❏ Mowing lawn (rider mower)
- ❏ Mowing lawn (power mower)
- ❏ Fishing in stream with waders
- ❏ Golf (power cart)
- ❏ Golf (walking, carrying, or pulling clubs)
- ❏ Mowing lawn (push mower)

WHERE ARE YOU NOW?

It is pretty easy to figure out which end of the physical activity continuum scale you are closer to. If your daily routine includes virtually no activities that would be classified as at least moderate-intensity, then it is probable that you would benefit from becoming more physically active. The key is to find an activity you enjoy—one that is right for you.

However, it is important not to beat yourself up about a sedentary lifestyle. In fact, a non-judgmental attitude can help you explore some of the reasons activity may not be part of your lifestyle. People avoid movement for many different reasons.

QUIZ: ARE YOU EXERCISE HESITANT?

Check any of the following that apply to you:

☐   I am positive I "should" be exercising.

☐   I am positive I need to exercise to look like society says I should.

☐   I have been pushed into exercise by others who had their own agenda; possibly, they wanted me to "have fun" or to lose weight.

☐   As a child, I felt pressure to perform in athletics.

☐   I have perfectionist tendencies and believe that "if I can't do it right, I won't do it at all."

☐   In the past, I typically exercised only when dieting. When I quit dieting, I usually quit exercising.

☐   I have been injured while exercising, and the whole idea of it scares me.

☐   I have exercised primarily as a way to lose weight.

☐   I was almost always the last one picked for team sports.

☐   If I miss a day or two of my exercise routine, I usually feel like I have blown it, and it is hard for me to get going again.

☐   I often feel intimidated by exercise, the equipment, or the fancy moves in aerobics.

☐   I often feel rejected by friends, family, or society because of the size or shape of my body.

☐   I feel bad about my body and on some level believe that the less I move, the less attention I call to my body.

☐   I think that others dislike my body, so I move less to call less attention to my body.

☐   I have used exercise as an external measure of self-worth.

☐   I have used exercise as a "punishment."

☐   I have forced myself to exercise when I ate too much or did not lose enough weight.

☐   I have been sexually abused at some time in my life.

Review the sentences you checked off. These can give you a clue to understanding why it may be difficult to connect with physical activity. Discussing these issues with a trusted friend can help your sort through some of the confusion. Sometimes this is enough to remove the barriers. In other cases, a skilled therapist can help you.

Source: Karin Kratina, Nancy King, and Dayle Hayes, *Moving Away From Diets: New Ways to Heal Eating Problems and Exercise Resistance*, 1996.

MY ACTIVITY LOG

To get a more accurate picture of your current activity level, try to fill out an activity log for one week. Make a photocopy of the next page and make sure you put it in a place where you will see it. Write down all the activities you do for one week.

ACTIVITY LOG

Time	Mon	Tues	Wed	Thurs	Fri	Sat	Sun
AM							
6–9							
9–12							
PM							
12–3							
3–6							
6–9							

Do not dwell on intensity. Just make a commitment to get moving at any speed. Try writing down ways you can add physical activity to your life (for ideas go to the next page).

Write down five ways you can get more movement into your life:

1. _____

2. _____

3. _____

4. _____

5. _____

15 WAYS TO LEAVE YOUR SOFA (AND GET MOVING)

1. At least twice a week, take an after-dinner walk with the whole family. One of the easiest ways to move more is to walk more!

2. Take your children to the local high-school track and let them play in the long-jump pit (which makes a great sandbox) while you walk a few laps with your spouse. You can keep an eye on them, and they can see their parents having fun walking and talking. Do it frequently, and one day your kids will pass along this behavior to your grandchildren.

3. Instead of telling your kids to "go out and play," ask them to "come out and play."

4. Walk around the house while talking on the phone—call them "frequent dialer" miles!

5. Bat a tennis ball back and forth with a friend.

6. Check out dance groups in your area. They love new dancers and are usually quite patient as you learn the fun steps.

7.   Do two minutes of stretching during a TV commercial break.

8.   Bowl, invite friends, and make it a party. Jump up and down when you score.

9.   Walk up and down the concourse during a layover at the airport.

10. When you get your morning newspaper, take a five-minute walk before going back inside the house.

11. Play catch or Frisbee with a friend—or your dog.

12. Take an extra walk around the mall perimeter when shopping.

13. Carry all the groceries from the car rather than ask for help, and flex your biceps as you carry each bag in.

14. Make a point of taking the stairs instead of the elevator; if you work in a high-rise office building, gradually add more flights.

15. Rake leaves, garden, or mow the lawn with a push mower.

PHYSICAL ACTIVITY: A "GATEWAY BEHAVIOR"

Physical activity is a "gateway behavior" to better health. Adopting a healthful behavior, such as becoming more physically active, tends to encourage the adoption of other more healthful choices. People who increase their physical activity level are more likely to eat healthy and are more likely to quit smoking.

MOVING UP THE PHYSICAL ACTIVITY CONTINUUM—IMPROVING FITNESS

So you have done it. You have added movement to your life and are accumulating roughly 30 minutes of moderate activity on most days of the week. And even on those days that you do not get at least 30 minutes, you are more active.

But now you may consider moving even further up the physical activity continuum into the range of fitness-related activity. This requires more effort, not necessarily in terms of time, but definitely in terms of intensity. Keep in mind that if you have made the transition to consistent moderate activity, you already have achieved most of the significant health benefits of an active lifestyle. And you will feel better, plus have more energy to do the things you have been wanting to do.

Adding more vigorous activity to your life may provide even more health benefits, but you will want to consider the following steps:

1. Make sure you are ready for it

2. Ease into it

3. Make sure it is enjoyable

4. Do not over-do it

PHYSICAL ACTIVITY READINESS QUESTIONNAIRE

This questionnaire is designed to help you help yourself. Many health benefits are associated with regular exercise, and completion of this worksheet is a sensible step to take if you are planning to increase the amount of physical activity in your life. For most people, physical activity should not pose any problem or hazard. This worksheet has been designed to identify the small number of adults for whom physical activity might be inappropriate, or those who have been given medical advice concerning the type of activity most suitable for them.

Common sense is your best guide in answering these few questions. Please read them carefully and check the "YES" or "NO" box opposite each question as it applies to you.

YES	NO	
		1. Has your doctor ever said you have heart trouble?
		2. Do you frequently have pains in your heart and chest?
		3. Do you often feel faint or have spells of severe dizziness?
		4. Has a doctor ever said your blood pressure was too high?
		5. Has your doctor ever told you that you have a bone or joint problem, such as arthritis, that has been aggravated by exercise or might be made worse with exercise?
		6. Is there a good physical reason not mentioned here why you should not follow an activity program even if you wanted to?
		7. Are you over age 65 and not accustomed to vigorous exercise?

If you answered:

YES TO ONE OR MORE QUESTIONS:

If you have not recently done so, consult with your physician by telephone or in person BEFORE increasing your physical activity and/or getting a fitness appraisal. Tell your physician what questions you answered YES to on this questionnaire.

After medical evaluation, seek advice from your physician as to your suitability for:

- Unrestricted physical activity—starting off easily and progressing gradually.

- Restricted or supervised activity to meet your specific needs, at least on an initial basis; check in your community for special programs or services.

NO TO ALL QUESTIONS:

If you answered the questionnaire accurately, you have reasonable assurance of your present suitability for:

- A graduated exercise program—a gradual increase in proper exercise promotes good fitness development while minimizing or eliminating discomfort.

- An exercise test—simple tests of fitness or more complex types may be undertaken, if you so desire.

Source: Developed by the British Columbia Ministry of Health. Conceptualized and critiqued by the Multidisciplinary Advisory Board on Exercise (MABE).

HOW PHYSICALLY FIT AM I?

You may be physically active, but are you physically fit? Physical fitness refers to three major components: aerobic fitness, muscular strength, and flexibility.

AEROBIC FITNESS

Aerobic fitness measures the strength and ability of your heart, lungs, circulation, and muscles to sustain vigorous activity. Aerobic activities speed your heart rate and breathing and help cardiovascular fitness, as well as reduce your risk of heart disease, type 2 diabetes, and certain cancers.

MUSCULAR STRENGTH

Muscular strength is important for overall physical function and quality of life. Most of us will lose significant amounts of muscle mass during our adult lives, and this can affect our quality of life, particularly beyond the age of 50. Regularly performing strengthening exercises may help build and maintain your bones and prevent muscle loss.

FLEXIBILITY

Flexibility is important because it increases our range of joint motion so we can enjoy many of our favorite activities. It allows us to move with less risk of injury to our joints and muscles.

AEROBIC FITNESS—HOW DO I MEASURE UP?

Follow the simple directions below to take the 12-minute walk/jog test.

Purpose: To measure the capacity of your lungs, cardiovascular system, and muscles to sustain vigorous exercise.

What you need:

- Indoor or outdoor track (almost all high schools have one).
- Stopwatch or watch with a second hand.
- Comfortable clothing and walking/jogging shoes.

Before the test:

- It is best not to have a heavy meal within a few hours of the test.
- Warm up by walking briskly or jogging for a few minutes, and then do some light stretching.

Procedures:

- Use the inside lane of a quarter-mile track and try to cover as much distance as you can in 12 minutes. Do not start out too fast, and try to maintain a constant pace. You may walk, jog, or run—or combine all three if you wish.

- After you finish, record how many laps you completed. If the last lap is not a complete lap, estimate it to the nearest tenth of a lap. Write the number here _____.
- Continue to walk slowly for a few minutes to allow your heart rate and blood pressure to return to normal levels.
- Use the chart below to assess your aerobic fitness level.

MEN

| Percentile Rank | Fitness Category | Age | | | | |
		20–29	30–39	40–49	50–59	60+
		Laps Completed				
80	Very High	>6.6	>6.4	>6.2	>5.8	>5.5
60	High	6.2	6.0	5.7	5.3	5.0
40	Moderate	5.8	5.6	5.3	5.0	4.6
20	Low	<5.4	<5.2	<4.9	<4.6	<4.2

WOMEN

| Percentile Rank | Fitness Category | Age | | | | |
		20–29	30–39	40–49	50–59	60+
		Laps Completed				
80	Very High	>5.8	>5.5	>5.3	>4.8	>4.7
60	High	5.3	5.1	4.8	4.5	4.3
40	Moderate	5.0	4.8	4.5	4.2	4.0
20	Low	<4.6	<4.4	<4.2	<3.9	<3.8

Source: Cooper Institute for Aerobics Research, Dallas, Texas.

HOW STRONG AM I?—PUSH-UP TEST FOR MUSCULAR STRENGTH AND ENDURANCE

Purpose: To measure strength and short-term endurance of the upper body muscles.

What you need:

- Stopwatch or watch with a second hand.

Before the test:

- Do some light stretching (especially stretch the shoulders).

Procedures:

- Kneel down on the floor and place your hands shoulder-width apart; arms should be fully extended, and fingers should be spread and pointed forward.
- Place a rolled-up or folded towel—about three to four inches thick—on the floor under your chest.
- Extend your feet out behind you and lift your knees so that your body weight is supported by your arms and toes; your back should be in a straight line with your legs.
- The push-up starts from the up-position; while keeping your back and legs in a straight line, bend your arms at the elbow to lower your chest so that it just touches the towel.
- Then push yourself back up to the starting position.
- Inhale on the way down; exhale on the way up.
- Complete as many push-ups as you can in one minute; write the number here _____.

(Modified push-up: For women who may have difficulty with the "full" push-up, keep your knees on the floor with your back and upper legs in a straight line. You may let your feet come up off the floor during the push-up.)

Use the chart below to assess your level of muscular strength and endurance.

WORKSHEET: HOW STRONG AM I?

MEN (FULL PUSH-UP)

Percentile Rank	Fitness Category	20–29	30–39	Age 40–49	50–59	60+
		Push-Ups Completed				
80	Very High	>47	>39	>30	>25	>23
60	High	37	30	24	19	18
40	Moderate	29	24	18	13	10
20	Low	<22	<17	<11	<9	<6

WOMEN (MODIFIED PUSH-UP)

Percentile Rank	Fitness Category	20–29	30–39	Age 40–49	50–59	60+
		Modified Push-Ups Completed				
80	Very High	>36	>31	>24	>21	>15
60	High	30	24	18	17	12
40	Moderate	23	19	13	12	5
20	Low	<11	<7	<6	<6	<2

WOMEN (FULL PUSH-UP)

Percentile Rank	Fitness Category	20–29	30–39	Age 40–49
		Push-Ups Completed		
80	Very High	>28	>23	>15
60	High	21	15	13
40	Moderate	15	11	9
20	Low	<10	<8	<6

Source: Cooper Institute for Aerobics Research, Dallas, Texas.

HOW FLEXIBLE AM I?—SIT AND REACH TEST FOR FLEXIBILITY

Purpose: To measure the flexibility of the lower back and hamstring muscles.

What you need:
- A 12-inch box and a yardstick.

Before the test:
- Place the box against a wall. Place a yardstick flat on top of the box so that the yardstick is parallel with the floor and perpendicular to one of the top edges of the box. Secure the yardstick (with tape) so that the 15-inch mark is flush with one of the top edges of the box (i.e., the first 15 inches of the yardstick should be sticking out beyond the top edge of the box; SEE ALSO first step in procedures, below).
- Warm up with some light stretching.

Procedures:
- In your stocking feet, sit on the floor with your legs extended

out in front of you and the bottoms of your feet firmly against the box, roughly 6 inches apart and right under the yardstick (which should be in line with your legs and pointing right at your belly button).

- With your hands together, lean forward slowly and reach as far along the yardstick as possible and hold the position for about a second; keep your legs straight and flat on the floor. It may help to exhale as you lean forward.
- Be careful not to bounce or lunge as you reach.
- Your score is the farthest point on the yardstick reached by the tips of your middle fingers together. Record here to the nearest 1/4 inch _____.
- Repeat the test twice more, and record here _____ _____.
- Take the best of the three scores, and write here _____.
- Use the chart below to assess your flexibility level.

MEN

Percentile Rank	Fitness Category	Age				
		20–29	30–39	40–49	50–59	60+
		Distance Reached (Inches)				
80	Very High	>20.5	>19.5	>18.5	>17.5	>17.25
60	High	18.5	17.5	16.25	15.5	14.5
40	Moderate	16.5	15.5	14.25	13.25	12.5
20	Low	<14.5	<13.0	<12.0	<10.5	<10.0

WOMEN

Percentile Rank	Fitness Category	Age				
		20–29	30–39	40–49	50–59	60+
		Distance Reached (Inches)				
80	Very High	>22.5	>21.5	>20.5	>20.25	>19.0
60	High	20.5	20.0	19.0	18.5	17.0
40	Moderate	19.25	18.25	17.25	16.75	15.5
20	Low	<17.0	<16.5	<15.0	<14.75	<13.0

Source: Cooper Institute for Aerobics Research, Dallas, Texas.

IMPROVING/MAINTAINING YOUR AEROBIC FITNESS

Accumulate approximately 30 minutes of vigorous activity at least three days a week.

IMPROVING/MAINTAINING YOUR MUSCULAR STRENGTH

To improve and maintain muscular strength, you will want to engage in resistance-type exercises two to three days per week. Strength exercises can be done at a fitness center or in your home, if you know how to perform the movements properly (see tips below). For each strength exercise, aim for between eight to 15 repetitions. At-home exercises can easily be performed with hand and ankle weights that can be purchased at most sporting-goods stores. You also can use water bottles or emptied milk jugs filled with water or sand. For best results, follow these guidelines:

- Start slowly and build up gradually; this may minimize any muscle soreness that can occur.

- Use light weights at first, making sure you can perform the movements properly.

- Perform strength exercises smoothly. Avoid jerky movements. Take about two to four seconds to lift or push the weight, hold the position for a second or so, and then take two to four seconds to lower the weight.

- Do not hold your breath while doing strength exercises. Just breathe normally. You may find it helpful to breathe out as you lift or push the weight, and breathe in as you reverse the movement.

IMPROVING/MAINTAINING YOUR FLEXIBILITY

Stretching can be done at almost any time or place. Improving your flexibility can give you more freedom of movement to do activities you enjoy, and also reduce risk of injuries. The American College of Sports Medicine recommends stretching two to three days per week.

For best stretching results, follow these guidelines:

- Do each stretching exercise two to three times per week.

- During each session, do each stretching exercise about four times.

- Perform "static" stretching by slowly stretching into the desired position (usually to the point of very mild discomfort—but not pain), then holding that position for 10 to 30 seconds. Relax for about five to 10 seconds and then repeat the stretch, trying to go a bit farther.

- Do not bounce or lunge when stretching because this may increase risk of injury.

- It's best to be warm while stretching. Do some light aerobic activity first, moving your arms and legs. Stretching after a hot shower or bath is a good idea.

CHAPTER SEVEN

Eating Healthy: In Your Home, On the Road, and At Your Favorite Restaurants

How can you ensure proper nutrition, maintain your natural weight, and still eat meals you enjoy? This chapter will show you how to put the Food Guide Pyramid into action with great-tasting recipes and serving ideas.

Taste is actually a bigger nutrition issue than many of us realize. There's a lot involved in why you prefer certain foods, including social, emotional, and physical factors. In any case, the foods you enjoy are likely the ones you eat most. And the more often you eat them, the more significant their nutritional impact on your overall health!

Flavor, variety, nutrition, and health can be a part of every meal. The following step-by-step suggestions show how to put the Food Guide Pyramid to work for you.

HOW TO ADD GRAINS, FRUITS, AND VEGETABLES TO MEALS

Evelyn Tribole, author of *Stealth Health*, recommends many ways to increase the nutrient value of your meals, some of which you may remember from Chapter 1. These tips will not only help you get at least the minimum number of daily servings of grains, fruits, and vegetables recommended by the Food Guide Pyramid, but also important nutrients and fiber to help reduce your risk of heart disease and cancer.

- Puree a vegetable and add it to a sauce, soup, or side dish—for example, add pureed cauliflower to a noodle casserole.

- Grate or chop vegetables into tiny specks—for instance, include carrots in clam chowder.

- Steam (or microwave) eggplant or zucchini and add it to spaghetti sauce. Use fun or interesting shape pastas, rather than regular spaghetti.

- Add frozen broccoli to boiling macaroni, then combine with cheese after cooking.

- Serve whole grain crackers, along with other crackers, with cheese or chili.

- Sauté vegetables in dry white wine. The alcohol content is removed, as long as the wine boils, and the vegetables have a nice flavor without the fat—pour over wild rice pilaf.

- Enjoy more fruit with a smoothie pick-me-up. Try low-fat milk or yogurt blended with a frozen banana, strawberries, or raspberries. Add some granola or toasted oat cereal. Kids especially love smoothies.

- Crumble graham crackers or sprinkle wheat germ over yogurt or ice cream.

- Replace one-third of all-purpose flour with whole-wheat flour when baking breads, muffins, biscuits, cookies, and brownies; try adding dried fruits to a recipe.

- Try whole-wheat hamburger buns, pitas, frozen waffles, and cereals; use whole-wheat hamburger buns for sloppy Joes or as a pizza crust.

- Grind up your favorite cereal or use wheat germ as part of the coating for meats, such as chicken, and even french toast.

- Experiment with new grains. Try cracked wheat, millet, or quinoa. Many mainstream supermarkets now carry them.

REDUCING FAT IN YOUR RECIPES

Chapter 2 also provided a number of tips for reducing fat in your diet to improve your health. Here we expand on those suggestions and provide helpful information on reducing fat in recipes to enhance the nutritional value of your meals.

- Start by experimenting with cutting fat by a third or a half. For example, if a recipe calls for 4 tablespoons of margarine, try 1 or 2 tablespoons. Reduce the oil in a muffin recipe from 1 cup to ¾ cup. Make a note of it and, if the muffins are good, try ⅔ cup the next time. This works well in quick bread recipes, too.

- In many semi-prepared mixes, such as preseasoned rice mixes or macaroni and cheese, simply omit the butter or margarine. If your recipes call for sautéing vegetables in oil or butter, try several tablespoons of water, broth, or wine. Then steam in a covered pot. Try flavoring with broth, skim milk, wine, or fruit juice, or adding extra herbs, spices, and vegetables.

- Like to make sauces? You do not have to start with a roux—a paste of fat and flour—or cornstarch. The goal of the roux is to avoid lumps. You can get the same results by slowly adding cold milk or fruit juice directly to the flour or cornstarch to eliminate fat. Once smoothly blended, stir the mixture constantly over medium heat until it comes to a boil. Then add herbs, spices, lemon juice, extracts, or sweeteners.

• Try skim or low-fat milk in place of whole milk. However, skim milk may not cut it in some recipes, especially those that call for cream. In that case, use evaporated skim milk. It is great in casseroles and quiches and can even be whipped when partially frozen.

COOKING WITH LOW-FAT DAIRY PRODUCTS

Dairy products are an excellent source of calcium and protein, so it is well worth your while to find ways to add them to your recipes. These days, it is becoming much easier to avoid saturated fat because of the variety of low- and non-fat dairy products on the market. Try some of the following ideas.

• Low- or no-fat plain yogurt works well as a substitute for sour cream and can be mixed with mayonnaise in dishes such as coleslaw, tuna, and potato salads. Be careful in heated dishes because yogurt tends to become watery. Try whisking some flour into the yogurt before cooking, or add yogurt to the cooked food after removing it from the heat.

• Try adding low-fat milk to pancakes, breads, soups, and sauces.

• Blend low-fat cottage cheese with several tablespoons of skim milk or yogurt until smooth to create a delicious base for vegetable dips. This also works in desserts. Cottage cheese also is a good replacement for ricotta cheese and sour cream in casseroles. Regular cottage cheese works somewhat better in cooking. Skim milk ricotta cheese has less fat and fewer calories than regular ricotta, but is higher in both than regular or low-fat cottage cheese.

- Experiment with low-fat processed cheeses. Generally, they are much lower in fat and work well in cooked sauces, sandwiches, casseroles, and omelets.

- Low-fat, low-cholesterol cheeses available in specialty shops and at deli counters are not always significantly lower in calories or fat than regular cheese. Imitation dairy products, such as imitation sour cream and cream cheese, are not necessarily healthful choices, because they often contain highly saturated fats, such as palm or coconut oils.

MAKING MORE HEALTHFUL RECIPES WITHOUT SACRIFICING TASTE

It is not only possible to learn to like the habits that keep you healthy, it is easy to do if you are willing to experiment a bit. Your palate can easily become accustomed to the taste of healthier foods, and you may even start to prefer them. Try to make a few changes in your own tried-and-true recipes, and have fun! When you realize the substantial health benefits that can be gained by adding or switching just a few ingredients, you may begin to realize how simple and exciting good nutrition is.

It may take some time to become adept at the art of adapting recipes to suit your health goals. Be prepared to encounter a few flops along with your many successes. When you have a triumph, don't forget to write down your alterations so you can do it again!

HEALTHFUL EATING WHEN DINING OUT

Whether it's a business meeting over lunch, dinner from a neighborhood carry-out, or a fast-food meal with the kids, dining out is part of our lives. We eat out because it's easy, quick, and fun. But is it healthful? It can be. You can choose meals that are nutrient-dense and contribute to good health while still enjoying your food.

Today, more people want healthful food choices when they eat out. Service-oriented restaurants will make an effort to please their customers and meet their requests so they will come back.

Tips for ordering wisely:

- Ask questions. Be assertive. After considering your own health goals, explain to the waiter or waitress what you need.

- If you are not that hungry, consider ordering an appetizer for the main course or sharing a main dish. Experiment with foods that are broiled, grilled, roasted, poached, or steamed.

- Check in with your body to see what you really want. If your body craves something sweet after dinner, consider sharing a rich dessert.

BEFORE ... AND AFTER: ADAPTING TRADITIONAL RECIPES

Enjoy this healthful and tasty adaptation of a traditional, rich carrot cake.

Original Carrot Cake
    1¼ cups oil
    1½ cups sugar
    3 eggs
    2 cups all-purpose flour

2 tsp. baking soda
½ tsp. salt
2½ tsp. cinnamon
1 tsp. ground cloves
¼ tsp. nutmeg
8-oz. can crushed pineapple
2 cups carrots, grated
1 cup pecans, coarsely chopped

Original Cream Cheese Frosting
1 cup cream cheese
½ cup icing sugar
½ tsp. white vanilla (you can use darker vanilla, but it creates a darker color)

Preheat oven to 350° F. Beat oil, sugar, and eggs in a small mixing bowl until well blended. Mix dry ingredients together in a large bowl. Add egg mixture to dry ingredients and mix well. Add pineapple, carrots, and pecans; mix well. Pour batter into a greased and floured 9-inch springform pan. Bake for 55 to 60 minutes or until toothpick inserted in center comes out clean.

For frosting, cream the cream cheese in a small bowl. Add remainder of frosting ingredients and blend well. Cover cooled cake with frosting.

Reduced-Fat Carrot Cake
2/3 cup oil
2/3 cup honey
3 eggs
1 cup all-purpose flour
2/3 cup whole wheat flour
2 tsp. baking soda

    1 Tbsp. cinnamon
    1 tsp. ground cloves
    ¼ tsp. nutmeg
    8-oz. can crushed pineapple
2½ cups carrots, grated
¾ cup pecans, coarsely chopped

Reduced-Fat Cream Cheese Frosting
    1 cup light cream cheese
    1/3 cup icing sugar
    ½ tsp. white vanilla

Bake and prepare as original recipe. Add whole wheat flour when adding all-purpose flour.

Source: Adapted from *Tailoring Your Tastes* by Linda Omichinski and Heather Wiebe Hildebrand, 1995.

BENEFITS OF MODIFIED VERSION

- Lower in fat: use of light cream cheese (no noticeable change in flavor!)

- Lower in sugar, but still sweet: honey may taste sweeter, especially when served in warm foods, requiring lesser amounts

- Moist: addition of honey and more carrots used

- More fiber: more carrots, use of whole wheat flour

Remember, if you plan to modify foods that will be eaten by your family as well as yourself, be sure your changes are minor ones. Just as you are making gradual, changes in your own eating habits, your family members will be changing their taste for food. Allow time for their tastes to adapt.

LOWER-FAT MENU SUGGESTIONS

Depending on your personal health goals, you may want to consider some of the following lower-fat menu suggestions—there are many other delicious choices too. Eating out for health does not mean you have to give up tasty foods, so bon appétit!

ITALIAN
Consider:
- Minestrone soup
- Pasta with a tomato-based sauce, or white or red clam sauce
- Cioppino
- Chicken cacciatore
- Ravioli or tortellini in tomato sauce
- Pizza with vegetable toppings
- Potato gnocchi in tomato sauce
- Baked polenta with a hint of cheese

CAJUN
Consider:
- Boiled crawfish or shrimp
- Creole and jambalaya dishes
- Boiled or grilled seafood
- Turkey or roast beef
- Po' Boy sandwiches
- White rice
- Red beans and rice

MEXICAN
Consider:
- Chicken enchilada or tostada

- Arroz con pollo
- Baked cornmeal tamale
- Burrito with black beans and chicken
- Frijoles a la charra or borracho beans
- Black beans and rice
- Salsa, pico de gallo, cilantro, jalapeño peppers

FAMILY STYLE

Consider:

- Single hamburger or grilled chicken breast on a bun
- Turkey or ham sandwich
- Broiled, baked, or grilled fish, chicken, or lean meat
- Salad with fresh vegetables, dressing on the side
- Baked potato with herbs
- Broth-based soups with lots of vegetables

FRENCH

Consider:

- Steamed mussels in tomato and wine sauce (use French bread to soak up the sauce)
- Mixed green salad with vinaigrette dressing
- Meats cooked in bordelaise or other wine-based sauce
- Lightly-sautéed, crisp vegetables
- Flambéed cherries in a crepe
- Peaches in wine

STEAKHOUSES

Consider:

- Leaner cuts of meat (London broil, filet mignon, round or flank steak, sirloin tip, tenderloin)
- Baked potato or rice
- Tossed green salad with dressing on the side
- Steamed vegetables

ASIAN

Consider:

- Wonton or hot and sour miso soup
- Steamed vegetable pot-stickers
- Dishes with lots of vegetables, water chestnuts
- Chicken, fish, or lean meat cooked in broth or steamed with vegetables
- Sushi or sashimi
- Teriyaki, sweet and sour, plum, or duck sauce
- Yakitori
- Steamed rice, dumpling, or noodle dishes
- Thai seafood stew
- Pho

GREEK AND MIDDLE EASTERN

Consider:

- Appetizers with rice or eggplant
- Dolmas (rice-stuffed grape leaves)
- Tzatziki (yogurt and cucumber appetizer) with pita
- Roast lamb, chicken, or lean beef shish kabob Couscous or bulgur wheat with vegetables or chicken
- Chicken pita sandwich
- Plaki (fish cooked in tomatoes, onions, and garlic)

INDIAN

Consider:

- Curries made with a vegetable or dal base
- Papadum or papad (crispy, thin lentil wafers)
- Chicken or beef tikka
- Chicken, beef, or fish tandoori
- Gobhi matar tamatar (cauliflower with peas and tomatoes)
- Matar pulau (rice pilaf with peas)
- Chicken saag (chicken with spinach) with steamed rice

- Chapati (thin, dry, whole-wheat bread) or naan (leavened bread topped with poppy seeds)

CAN FAST FOOD BE HEALTHY?

If you are like most people, you probably enjoy the convenience of eating at a fast-food restaurant every now and then. But you also may wonder if it's possible to choose healthful foods at a fast-food restaurant. It is!

How? Consider, for example, that orange juice has vitamin C and folic acid. Chili and salad offer fiber. Baked potatoes and vegetables provide vitamins and minerals. Grilled chicken and red meat are good sources of iron and protein. Breads offer B vitamins, including folic acid. Low-fat milk, reduced-fat shakes, and frozen yogurt are rich in calcium.

Although selections will vary from one restaurant to the next, the following tips can help you choose a meal that's tasty, relatively low in fat, and also provides a good supply of nutrients.

- If you're having fast food for one meal, let your other meals that day be based around fruits, vegetables, and grain foods to ensure you are getting enough nutrients from the Food Guide Pyramid throughout the entire day.

- Think about how your food will be cooked. Baked or broiled chicken and fish are more nutrient dense—less so if they are breaded and deep fried.

- If breakfast is your fast-food meal, consider a bagel with low-fat cream cheese, toast, or English muffin. Adding fruit juice or low-fat/skim milk can enhance the nutrient value of your meal.

BACK TO THE KITCHEN

Now that you may be less hesitant to alter recipes and shop for health, let's have some fun in the kitchen. These recipes have already been altered to enhance nutritional value and taste-tested, and are ready for your enjoyment. Remember, your body will tell you how much to eat!

BREAKFAST RECIPES

- Cracked Wheat Cereal
- Breakfast Couscous
- Quick All-Purpose Mix
- Quick-Mix Pancakes
- Quick-Mix Biscuits
- Quick-Mix Coffeecake

Cracked-Wheat Cereal

This recipe is easy to prepare, but takes a bit of time to cook and is worth it!

1/3 cup cracked wheat
2/3 cup water
1 cup low-fat milk
1 tsp. ground cinnamon
¼ cup raisins

Place the cracked wheat and ⅔ cup of water in a heavy-bottomed saucepan. Boil for 10 minutes. Add the milk and cinnamon. Reduce the heat to low. Cook for 30 minutes, until the cereal is creamy. Stir in the raisins.

Makes 1 serving.

Source: Estrogen the Natural Way, by Nina Shandler, 1997

Breakfast Couscous
>   2 cups 1% milk, hot
>   1 cup couscous
>   1 cup raisins, soaked in water and drained
>   Honey, to taste

Add couscous to hot milk and let stand 5 minutes. Stir in raisins and honey, to taste.

Makes 4 servings.

Source: Wheat Foods Council

Quick All-Purpose Mix
This all-purpose mix is great for making the pancakes, biscuits, and coffeecake shown below, as well as waffles or muffins.
>   8 cups whole wheat or all-purpose flour, or a combination
>   1 Tbsp. salt (or to taste)
>   1 cup instant dry milk
>   1/3 cup baking powder
>   2½ cups wheat germ

Mix thoroughly and store in a tightly covered jar in the refrigerator.

Source: Adapted from *Diet From a Small Planet,* by Frances Moore Lappe, 1982

Quick Mix Pancakes
>   1 egg
>   1 cup low-fat milk, buttermilk, or yogurt
>   3 Tbsp. oil
>   1½ cups Quick All-Purpose Mix

Beat egg and combine with milk and oil. Stir in mix and fry on a griddle.

Makes approximately 8 servings.

Source: Adapted from *Diet From a Small Planet,* by Frances Moore Lappe, 1982

Quick-Mix Biscuits

    1/3 cup oil or melted margarine

    2/3 cup low-fat milk, buttermilk, or low-fat yogurt

    2¼ cups Quick All-Purpose Mix

Preheat oven to 450°F. Combine oil and milk and stir in mix. Turn out onto a floured board and knead lightly. Pat or roll out 1-inch thick, cut with a biscuit cutter, and place on a greased baking sheet. Bake for 12 to 15 minutes.

Makes 16 biscuits.

Source: Adapted from *Diet From a Small Planet*, by Frances Moore Lappe, 1982

Quick-Mix Coffeecake

    1 egg

    ¼ cup oil plus 1 Tbsp.

    ¾ cup low-fat milk, buttermilk, or low-fat yogurt

    ¾ cup tightly packed brown sugar

    1½ cups Quick All-Purpose Mix

    1½ tsp. cinnamon Dried fruit (optional)

    ½ cup nuts (optional)

    ½ cup shredded coconut (optional)

Preheat oven to 375°F. Beat egg and combine with ¼ cup oil, milk, and ½ cup brown sugar. Stir in mix and dried fruit. Combine cinnamon, remaining ¼ cup brown sugar and 1 tablespoon oil, nuts, and coconut. Sprinkle crumbly mixture over batter and bake for 30 minutes.

Makes approximately 8 servings.

Source: Adapted from *Diet From a Small Planet*, by Frances Moore Lappe, 1982

SNACK RECIPES

- Banana Whole Wheat Muffins
- Southwest Salsa and Chili Pita Chips
- Yogurt-Bran Muffins
- Roasted Red-Pepper Dip

Banana Whole Wheat Muffins

    2 to 3 large ripe bananas, mashed (1½ cups)
    ½ cup honey
    4 Tbsp. low-fat plain yogurt
    2 tsp. cinnamon
    ¾ tsp. ground nutmeg
    ½ tsp. ground coriander
    1 large egg
    3 large egg whites
    1½ tsp. vanilla extract
    1 cup whole wheat flour
    1 1/4 cup all-purpose flour
    1 tbsp. baking soda
    1 tsp. baking powder
    ½ cup lightly toasted walnuts, chopped

Preheat oven to 350°F. Whisk together first 9 ingredients (bananas through vanilla extract) in a large mixing bowl. In a separate bowl, whisk together the flours, baking soda, and baking powder. Add all at once to banana mixture, mixing with a spatula, just until blended. Stir in nuts. Lightly coat muffin tins with cooking spray. Fill muffin tins two-thirds full with batter. Bake for 18 to 20 minutes, or until a toothpick inserted into the center comes out clean. Remove pan from oven and allow to cool for a few minutes before removing muffins from pan. Cool muffins on a wire rack.

Makes 18 muffins.

Source: The Vegetarian Gourmet, by Florence and Mickey Bienenfeld, 1987

Southwest Salsa and Chili Pita Chips

Chili Pita Chips

6 – 5½-inch white or whole wheat pita bread pockets

3 Tbsp. olive oil

Chili powder to season

Preheat oven to 350°F. Split each pita bread horizontally into 2 rounds. Lightly brush the rough sides with the olive oil. Lightly sprinkle chili powder over the surfaces. Cut each pita round into wedges. Arrange the triangles on a baking sheet and bake for 5 to 10 minutes, or until lightly toasted. Serve with Southwest Salsa or use as an accompaniment with soups and salads. Store leftover chips in an airtight container at room temperature up to five days.

Salsa

3 cups chopped tomatoes

½ cup chopped fresh cilantro

½ cup chopped red onion

½ cup cooked corn, fresh or frozen and thawed

½ cup cooked black beans or canned black beans, drained and rinsed

1 jalapeño pepper (optional), seeded and finely chopped

Juice of one lime (about ¼ cup)

¼ tsp. salt

In a large bowl, combine all ingredients; mix well.

Makes approximately 72 chips and 3 cups of salsa.

Source: Wheat Foods Council

Yogurt-Bran Muffins

  ½ cup boiling water
  ½ cup bran cereal
  2/3 cup packed brown sugar
  ¼ cup applesauce
  1 egg, slightly beaten
  1 cup low-fat vanilla yogurt
  1 cup all-bran cereal
  ½ cup whole wheat flour
  1 cup cake flour
  1¼ tsp. baking soda
  ½ tsp. salt
  1 tsp. baking powder
  Nonstick cooking spray

In a small bowl, pour boiling water over the bran cereal. Set aside and let stand. In a large bowl, combine the brown sugar, applesauce, beaten egg, low-fat yogurt, and all-bran cereal; mix well. Sift whole wheat flour, cake flour, baking soda, salt, and baking powder together; mix with the above ingredients. Mix bran cereal into other ingredients; mix well. Spray a muffin pan with cooking spray and fill each cup with ¼ cup of batter. Bake in a 400°F preheated oven for 10 minutes.

Makes 12 muffins.

Source: Wheat Foods Council

Roasted Red Pepper Dip

  8 oz. nonfat sour cream
  1 7-oz. jar roasted red peppers, drained
  4 oz. nonfat cream cheese
  1 clove garlic
  1 Tbsp. fresh basil leaves
  ½ Tbsp. dried oregano leaves

64 fat-free wheat crackers

In a food processor or electric blender, add all ingredients except crackers. Process just until red peppers are finely chopped. Pour into bowl. Chill at least 1 hour. Serve with crackers.

Makes approximately 2 cups.
Source: Wheat Foods Council

LUNCH/DINNER RECIPES

- Southwest Pasta Salad
- Tortilla Roll-Ups
- Sun-Dried Tomato and Walnuts Tossed With Penne Pasta
- Chili Relleno Casserole
- Cheese Sauce for Veggies

Southwest Pasta Salad

12 oz. tri-color rotini
1 11-oz. can whole kernel corn, drained
1/3 cup chopped red-pepper
1/3 cup chopped green pepper
1 15-oz. can kidney beans, drained and rinsed
3 green onions, chopped
1 cup oil-free salad dressing
2 to 3 Tbsp. salad seasoning
¾ cup grated cheddar cheese

Prepare pasta according to package directions; rinse with cold water and drain. In a large bowl, combine pasta, corn, red and green peppers, kidney beans, and onion. Mix salad dressing with salad seasoning and add to pasta mixture. Add cheese and toss. Refrigerate 3 to 4 hours to allow flavors to blend. Add additional salad dressing if desired.

Makes approximately 6 servings.
Source: Wheat Foods Council

Tortilla Roll-Ups

    4 10-inch flour tortillas

    2 Tbsp. low-fat salad dressing or mayonnaise

    ½ cup chunky salsa

    4 oz. sliced smoked turkey or roast beef

    1/3 cup shredded low-fat cheddar cheese

    ½ cup thin strips red-pepper

    ½ cup sliced green onions

    2 Tbsp. sliced black olives

Spread salad dressing on tortilla; spread salsa over salad dressing. Top with meat, cheese, and vegetables as desired. Roll up and serve, or heat 1 minute in microwave on medium power. Each tortilla may be wrapped in plastic wrap after rolling and then refrigerated. For bite-sized snacks, cut in 1-inch slices.

Makes approximately 8 servings.

Source: Wheat Foods Council

Sun-Dried Tomato and Walnuts Tossed With Penne Pasta

    8 oz. penne pasta

    2 garlic cloves, pressed

    1/3 cup chopped walnuts, lightly toasted

    ¾ cup minced, bottled, sun-dried tomatoes, drained

    2 Tbsp. flax oil or other vegetable oil

    1 tsp. basil

    ½ cake (8 oz.) extra-firm tofu

    Salt, to taste

In a large saucepan, bring 3 quarts of water to a boil. Add the penne pasta and cook according to package directions. As the pasta cooks, prepare the sauce. Place the pressed garlic in a large bowl. Add the walnuts, sun-dried tomatoes, oil, and basil. Mash in the tofu and mix well with a spoon. When the pasta is ready, drain, and add it to the large bowl. Toss all ingredients until pasta is well-coated. Pour onto a platter and serve at room temperature or chilled.

Makes approximately 4 servings.

Source: Estrogen the Natural Way, by Nina Shandler, 1997

Chile Relleno Casserole

    Vegetable oil cooking spray
    1 cup evaporated skim milk
    4 egg whites
    1/3 cup all-purpose flour
    3 4-oz. cans whole green chilies
    ½ lb. low-fat jack cheese, grated
    ½ lb. low-fat sharp cheddar cheese, grated
    1 8-oz. can tomato sauce

Preheat oven to 350°F. Spray a deep 1½-quart casserole dish with vegetable oil cooking spray. Beat evaporated skim milk, egg whites, and flour together until smooth. Split open chilies and rinse to remove seeds; drain on a paper towel. Mix cheeses together and reserve ½ cup for topping. Alternate layers of chilies, cheese, and egg mixture in casserole dish. Pour tomato sauce over top layer and sprinkle with reserved cheese. Bake one hour or until done in the center.

Makes approximately 8 servings.

Source: Shape Magazine's "Recipe Makeover," by Evelyn Tribole, April 1991

Cheese Sauce for Vegetables

    ¼ cup white wine
    ¼ cup Spanish onion, minced
    1 clove garlic, minced
    2 Tbsp. all-purpose or whole wheat flour
    1 cup 1% milk

    1 tsp. caraway seed
    1/8 tsp. pepper
    ½ cup cheddar or Swiss cheese
    ¼ cup part-skim mozzarella cheese

Sauté onions and garlic in the white wine in a non-stick pan. Sprinkle flour over the hot onions and garlic, stirring constantly. Cook for about 1 minute. Add milk to hot ingredients in pan and whisk ingredients together. Cook until it starts to thicken, stirring frequently. Add spices and grated cheese to the milk mixture. Continue to heat until the mixture is hot. Serve immediately over hot steamed vegetables.

Makes approximately 8 servings.

Source: Tailoring Your Tastes, by Linda Omichinski and Heather Wiebe Hildebrand, 1995

DESSERT RECIPES

- Healthy Date-Nut Cookies
- Golden Pound Cake
- Old-Fashioned Bread Pudding

Healthy Date-Nut Cookies
    1 cup pecans
    1 cup dates (or ½ cup dates and ½ cup raisins)
    2 egg whites, beaten
    4 egg whites, beaten
    2 Tbsp. honey
    1 tsp. vanilla
    1 tsp. cinnamon
    ½ cup whole wheat flour
    ½ tsp. baking powder

Preheat oven to 350°F. Chop pecans in a blender or food processor. Blend in dates and 2 egg whites until dates are well mashed. Place date mixture in a large mixing bowl and set aside. Beat 4 egg whites in an electric mixer until foamy. Gradually beat in honey and vanilla; continue beating until whites are thick and shiny. Mix together cinnamon, flour, and baking powder. Reduce speed and lightly fold dry ingredients into whites. Stir ½ of the egg-white mixture into the date mixture, then carefully fold in the remaining egg-white mixture. Drop by spoonfuls onto two nonstick cookie sheets and bake for approximately 20 minutes or until light brown.

Makes 30 to 36 cookies.

Source: The Vegetarian Gourmet, by Florence and Mickey Bienenfeld, 1987

Golden Pound Cake

    2½ cups cake flour, plus 1 tsp. for pan preparation
    2/3 cup sugar
    ½ cup margarine (1 stick), softened
    3 egg whites
    2 tsp. vanilla extract
    1 tsp. almond extract
    1 tsp. lemon extract
    1 tsp. baking soda
    ¼ tsp. salt
    8 oz. low-fat lemon yogurt
    Butter-flavored vegetable cooking spray

Prepare 8½- x 4½- x 3-inch loaf pan with cooking spray and dust with 1 tsp. of flour. In a mixing bowl, cream sugar and margarine at medium speed with electric mixer until fluffy. Add egg whites and continue beating at medium speed for 3 to 4 minutes, or until well blended. Add vanilla, almond, and lemon extracts, blending at low speed until well mixed. In another bowl, combine sifted flour, baking soda, and salt. Alternately add the flour and yogurt to the mixture, blending completely after each addition. (Begin and end with flour additions.) Pour batter into prepared loaf pan and bake at 350°F for 1 hour, or until toothpick comes out clean. Cool in pan for 10 minutes, then remove from pan to cooling rack. Cut loaf into 16 slices and serve plain or top with fruit.

Makes approximately 16 servings.
Source: Wheat Foods Council

Old-Fashioned Bread Pudding

This is good for using up old bread or dried-out cake. You can use left-over banana bread, corn bread (plain, not the onion and cheese kind), carrot cake, gingerbread—whatever lends itself to your taste. This recipe is geared for regular, unsweet bread. If you do use cake or sweet bread, adjust the amounts of sweetening, spice, and vanilla to taste.

Preheat oven to 350°F. In a large bowl, beat the following ingredients together well (you can use a blender).
   3 cups milk
   3 eggs (large)
   ½ tsp. salt
   ½ tsp. cinnamon
   Juice from ½ lemon
   2 tsp. vanilla extract
   3 Tbsp. honey
   2 Tbsp. sugar

Mix together in a 9- x 13-inch baking pan: 4 cups coarsely crumbled bread, 1½ cups freshly grated apple and/or ½ cup chopped, dried fruit ½ cup chopped nuts (optional)

Pour the first mixture into the pan and push everything around with a wooden spoon until it is uniformly combined. Bake 35 minutes. Serve hot, warm, or cold with heavy cream, ice cream, applesauce, or fresh fruit.

Makes approximately 12 servings.

Source: The Moosewood Cookbook, by Mollie Katzen, 1977

CHAPTER EIGHT

Making It All Work

HOW DO YOU GET STARTED ON THE PATH TO BETTER HEALTH? HOW DO YOU STAY MOTIVATED ONCE YOU ARE THERE? THIS CHAPTER WILL HELP YOU INTEGRATE THE CHANGES DISCUSSED IN THIS BOOK INTO YOUR LIFESTYLE.

AFTER HAVING READ this book so far, you may be asking, "But how can I make it all work?" Change, as we all know, is easier said than done. Most of us would like to make positive changes in our lives: being more productive at work; spending more quality time with family; or taking better care of our health. The process of change, however, is quite challenging.

If modifying our behavior was so easy, we would not have to keep making New Year's resolutions each year—sometimes the same resolutions again and again. How many times have you resolved to lose weight? To improve your diet? Or to exercise more? Why is it so difficult to maintain the changes we make?

As you strive to make healthful eating and regular physical activity a permanent part of your life, you will pass through all—or some—of the five stages outlined by psychologist James O. Prochaska, Ph.D., originator of the Transtheoretical Model of behavior change. Take a look and see where you are at right now!

STAGES OF CHANGE

STAGE 1: PRECONTEMPLATION

Lack of information is the key marker of this stage. You may not have heard of the Food Guide Pyramid and probably are unaware of all the health benefits of leading a physically active lifestyle. Without this knowledge, you do not see the need for lifestyle changes that may enhance the quality of your life.

Chances are, you are beyond the precontemplation stage—especially because reading this book means you now have information on the many benefits of healthful eating and physical activity.

STAGE 2: CONTEMPLATION

You are thinking about making lifestyle changes and becoming more active, but you do not know exactly where to start. You may feel like you have been bombarded with information on nutrition and fitness from the media and are confused. One of the reasons for writing this book was to set the record straight regarding nutrition and exercise and to provide straightforward information to allow you to make positive changes in your life.

STAGE 3: PREPARATION

You may not have changed any aspect of what you eat yet, and you may not have become more physically active. But you have moved beyond just thinking about change—you have formulated a plan and are ready to take action.

You have completed the quizzes and questionnaires in the previous chapters. You have made lists of things you can do to improve your health, change the way you view food, and become more physically active. You are aware of where you are now and have a good idea of where you are going and how to get there. You are ready for action!

Stage 4: Action

This is the exciting part—changing! We suggest you copy a picture of the Food Guide Pyramid from this book and tape it to your refrigerator. It can serve as a constant reminder.

You can decide for yourself just what changes you feel comfortable making first. You may wish to focus on improving your nutrition and not even think about physical activity. If you are on the right track, nutrition-wise, then you may want to start by taking steps to be more active.

If you make small changes and build on them, your chances of success are much better. Most people will be able to see results in a matter of weeks. You will probably notice more energy, improved stamina, and an overall improved sense of well-being. Just knowing you are taking charge of your health can be empowering.

Stage 5: Maintenance

The changes you have made in nutrition and physical activity are now a routine part of your life—as routine as bathing, combing your hair, and brushing your teeth. It may be helpful to redo some of the worksheets in this book and compare how you are doing after a few weeks or months.

Do not let past experiences discourage you or hold you back. You may have started an exercise program before, but did not stick with it, perhaps, because the approach or timing was not right for you.

Perhaps the exercise program focused more on weight loss rather than enjoyable physical activity. Again, if you make small changes, and build on them, your chances of success are much better. Also, focus on the process—the satisfaction of eating well and the fun of an active lifestyle—rather than an arbitrary end point dictated by numbers on the scale.

THE IMPORTANCE OF FEEDBACK

We often interpret vital, constructive feedback—whether from our bodies, our minds, or our friends—as criticism and judgment. Yet, feedback is critical for us to stay on target with our health goals.

Feedback can take many forms:

- How your body feels when you eat—or think you eat—too much

- How your body feels when you eat too little

- How your body feels when you do not get any physical activity

- How your body feels when you are getting enough physical activity

- Writing down on a piece of paper the foods you eat to see if you are meeting the Food Guide Pyramid minimums

- Paying attention to your internal cues of hunger and satiety

- Paying attention when a friend says he or she is concerned about you

You can use all these forms of feedback to keep you on track. If you overeat to the point of feeling stuffed at one meal, you have to trust your body to take appropriate action at the next meal, or the next day. Usually your internal cues will do this for you naturally. Occasional overeating is a part of normal eating, as is returning to listening to your body and letting your body tell you how much you need to eat.

Knowing whether you are getting enough fiber cannot be gauged by any internal mechanism—your body has no way of keeping a tally on the fiber you consume. If you eat according to the Food Guide Pyramid, you will not have to keep a tally.

Situations may arise—work schedule, vacation, travel, weather, illness—that upset your routine. You may find it difficult to eat like you are accustomed to or to squeeze in your usual physical activities. Not to worry—most of these routine-altering situations are temporary. Missing out on physical activity for a week is not the end of the world. Going without your favorite homemade cooking or traveling for business, can be viewed as opportunities to enjoy new dining experiences.

One of the biggest obstacles you may face is the frustration of not seeing results for quite a while. It's easy to set unrealistic expectations, and the first step to success is to be realistic about what you can accomplish and to face the fact that making a significant lifestyle change is a hard—though not impossible—task. Try these techniques for staying motivated when you seem to be fighting an uphill battle.

KEEP A POSITIVE ATTITUDE

Beating yourself up or feeling guilty about your health habits can sabotage your efforts to change before you get started. Be gentle with yourself, and remember, change is a matter of progress, not perfection. There is much to be said for self-acceptance. Change is always easier when you feel good about yourself.

> "When we accept ourselves as we are today and gradually proceed to make the changes we want for ourselves, we have more power to re-create our lives. When we are self-accepting, we love ourselves for not being perfect already. The burden of self-rejection makes it very hard to change our lives."
>
> – *Amrit Desai*

TAKE JUST ONE STEP

It is easy to get discouraged if you have resolved to make radical changes in every part of your life. Do not overwhelm yourself! Pick one main thing to change at a time, rather than adopting an all-or-nothing philosophy. Your accomplishments will be easier to see. Once you have been victorious in one area, you will feel more confident and better equipped to conquer new areas of wellness in your life.

BE NEAR-SIGHTED

The long-term benefits of exercising and eating healthy are clear. Many people tend to look for distant results, like a drop in weight or cholesterol level, and then get discouraged because they do not see change right away. Remember to focus on positive changes in your life in the here and now—like being in a better mood, having more energy to do the things you want to do, and experiencing less tension at work.

YOUR BEHAVIOR CHANGE CONTRACT

To help you achieve and maintain your own personal goals, we suggest you complete a behavior change contract. Writing down your goals, and the specific actions you intend to take to achieve those goals, is an important part of change. Sign and date the contract and be sure to get a witness to co-sign. The co-signer can serve as a source of encouragement and positive reinforcement. Post the contract in a place where you will always see it. Making just one change can have a significant impact on your overall health and wellness!

Make the actions easy to tally, as in the example below:

WORKSHEET: BEHAVIOR CHANGE CONTRACT EXAMPLE

Name: Sarah Smith

Concern: Things have been so hectic lately, I don't seem to be able to do the things I would like to do for my health.

Goal: Begin to take charge of my health by doing some minimal changes. Affirm to myself that small changes add up.

I will take these actions to work towards my goal:

1. Eat a minimum of 2 fruits or vegetables/day.
2. Do 3 - 5 min activity sessions/day.
3. Try peanut butter on a banana to see if it will help me enjoy the banana more 1 time.
4. Spend 10 mins each day relaxing with the novel I got last week.
5. Say affirmation daily "These small changes will add up to improved health and more energy."

Mark the box when the above actions are accomplished to check your progress toward your goal!

	Day 1	Day 2	Day 3	Day 4	Day 5	Day 6	Day 7
1	✓		✓	✓	✓		✓
2	✓	✓	✓	✓	✓	✓	
3			✓				
4	✓		✓	✓			✓
5	✓	✓	✓	✓	✓	✓	✓

I have established a goal and will take constructive actions to reach my goal. I am committed to follow through with this plan for the next seven days.

Sarah Smith
_____
Signature

_5 - 15 - 2000_
_____
Date

_____
Co-signed

_____
Date

WORKSHEET: BEHAVIOR CHANGE CONTRACT

Name:_____

Concern: _____

Goal: _____

I will take these actions to work towards my goal:

1. _____

2. _____

3. _____

4. _____

5. _____

Mark the box when the above actions are accomplished to check your progress toward your goal!

	Day 1	Day 2	Day 3	Day 4	Day 5	Day 6	Day 7
1							
2							
3							
4							
5							

I have established a goal and will take constructive actions to reach my goal. I am committed to follow through with this plan for the next seven days.

_____   _____
Signature   Co-signed

_____   _____
Date   Date

SOME FINAL ADVICE ...

- Be realistic

- Make small changes over time in what you eat; after all, small steps often work better than giant leaps

- Be adventurous

- Expand your tastes to enjoy a variety of foods

- Be flexible

- Go ahead and balance what you eat and the physical activity you do over several days—your body will work with you on this

- Be sensible

- Enjoy all foods and, if you listen and respond to your body's signals of hunger and satiety, you will not overdo it

- Be active

- Walk the dog, don't just watch the dog walk. You will feel good and have more energy too.

APPENDIX A

Food, Health, and Nutrition Organizations

AMERICAN CANCER SOCIETY
1599 Clifton Road Atlanta, GA 30329 Phone: (800) ACS-2345
http://www.cancer.org/

AMERICAN COLLEGE OF SPORTS MEDICINE
401 West Michigan Street Indianapolis, IN 46202 Phone: (317)
637-9200 *http://www.acsm.org/*

AMERICAN DIABETES ASSOCIATION
1701 North Beauregard Street Alexandria, VA 22311 Phone: (800)
DIABETES (342-2383); (800) 342-2383 *http://www.diabetes.org/*

AMERICAN DIETETIC ASSOCIATION
216 West Jackson Boulevard Chicago, IL 60606-6995 Phone: (312)
899-0040 *http://www.eatright.org/*

AMERICAN HEART ASSOCIATION
7272 Greenville Avenue Dallas, TX 75231 Phone: (214) 373-6300;
(800) AHA-USA1 *http://www.americanheart.org*

AMERICAN INSTITUTE FOR CANCER RESEARCH
1759 R Street, N.W. Washington, D.C. 20009 Phone: (800)
843-8114; (202) 328-7744 (in D.C.) Fax: (202) 328-7226 *http://
www.aicr.org* E-mail: *aicrweb@aicr.org*

AMERICAN MEDICAL ASSOCIATION
515 North State Street Chicago, IL 60610 Phone: (312) 464-5000
http://www.ama-assn.org/

AMERICAN PUBLIC HEALTH ASSOCIATION
800 I Street, N.W. Washington, D.C. 20001 Phone: (202) 777-
2742 (APHA) TTY: (202) 777-2500 Fax: (202) 777-2534 *http:
//www.apha.org*

AMERICAN RUNNING ASSOCIATION
4405 East West Highway, Suite 405 Bethesda, MD 20814 Phone:
(301) 913-9517; (800) 776-2732 Fax: (301) 913-9520 *http://
www.americanrunning.org/*

AMERICAN SOCIETY OF CLINICAL NUTRITION
9650 Rockville Pike Bethesda, MD 20814-3998 Phone: (301) 530-
7110 Fax: (301) 571-1863 *http://www.faseb.org/ascn/*

AMERICAN SCHOOL FOOD SERVICE ASSOCIATION
(ASFSA)
700 South Washington Street, Suite 300 Alexandria, VA 22314
Phone: (703) 739-3900 Fax: (703) 739-3915 *http://www.asfsa.org*

CANCER RESEARCH FOUNDATION
1600 Duke Street, Suite 110 Alexandria, VA 22314 Phone:
(703) 836-4412; (800) 227-CRFA Fax: (703) 836-4413 *http://
www.preventcancer.org/*

CELIAC SPRUE ASSOCIATION/USA, INC.
P.O. Box 31700 Omaha, NE 68131-0700 Phone: (402) 558-0600
Fax: (402) 558-1347

FOOD ALLERGY NETWORK
10400 Eaton Place, Suite 107 Fairfax, VA 22030-2208 Phone: (800) 929-4040 *http://www.foodallergy.org/*

FOOD MARKETING INSTITUTE
655 15th Street, N.W. Washington, D.C. 20005 Phone: (202) 452-8444 Fax: (202) 429-4519 *http://www.fmi.org* E-mail: *fmi@fmi.org*

INTERNATIONAL ASSOCIATION OF FITNESS PROFESSIONALS
6190 Cornerstone Court East, Suite 204 San Diego, CA 92121 Phone: (800) 999-4332; (858) 535-8979 Fax: (858) 535-8234 *http://www.ideafit.com/*

INTERNATIONAL FOOD INFORMATION COUNCIL FOUNDATION
1100 Connecticut Avenue, N.W., Suite 430 Washington, D.C. 20036 Phone: (202) 296-6540 Fax: (202) 296-6547 *http://ificinfo.health.org/* E-mail: *foodinfo@ific.health.org*

INSTITUTE OF FOOD TECHNOLOGISTS
221 North LaSalle Street, Suite 300 Chicago, IL 60601-1291 Phone: (312) 782-8424 Fax: (312) 782-8348 *http://www.ift.org* E-mail: *info@ift.org*

NATIONAL ASSOCIATION OF ANOREXIA NERVOSA AND ASSOCIATED DISORDERS
P.O. Box 7 Highland Park, IL 60035 Phone: (847) 831-3438 Fax: (847) 433-4632 *http://www.anad.org/* E-mail: *info@anad.org*

NATIONAL ACADEMY OF SCIENCES
Institute of Medicine Food & Nutrition Board 2101 Constitution
Avenue, N.W. Washington, D.C. 20418 Phone: (202) 334-2000
http://www.nas.edu/

NATIONAL CATTLEMEN'S BEEF ASSOCIATION
9110 East Nichols Avenue, Centennial, CO 80112
Phone: (303)220-9890 Fax: (303)220-9280 *http://
www.beefnutrition.org*

NATIONAL DAIRY COUNCIL
10255 West Higgins Road, Suite 900 Rosemont, IL 60018 Phone:
(847) 803-2000 Fax: (847) 803-2077 *http://www.nationaldairycounc
il.org/* E-mail: *ndc@bsmg.com*

NATIONAL DIABETES INFORMATION CLEARING-
HOUSE (NDIC)
1 Information Way Bethesda, MD 20892-3560 Phone: (301)
654-3327 Fax: (301) 907-8906 *http://www.niddk.nih.gov* E-mail:
ndic@info.niddk.nih.gov

NATIONAL MENTAL HEALTH ASSOCIATION
1201 Prince Street Alexandria, VA 22314-2971 Phone: (703)
684-7722 Fax: (703) 684-5968 Mental Health Information Center Phone: (800) 969-NMHA TTY: (800) 433-5959 *http://
www.nmha.org*

NATIONAL OSTEOPOROSIS FOUNDATION
1150 17th Street, N.W., Suite 500 Washington, D.C. 20036 Phone:
(202) 223-2226; (800) 223-9994 *http://www.nof.org*

NATIONAL PORK PRODUCERS COUNCIL
P.O. Box 10383 Des Moines, IA 50306 Phone: (515) 223-2600 Fax:
(515) 223-2646 *http://www.nppc.org/* E-mail: *pork@nppc.org*

NATIONAL RESTAURANT ASSOCIATION
1200 17th Street, N.W. Washington, D.C. 20036-3097 Phone:
(202) 331-5900 *http://www.restaurant.org/* E-mail: *info@dineout.org*

NATIONAL SUNFLOWER ASSOCIATION
4023 State Street Bismarck, ND 58501-0690 Phone: (701)
328-5100; (888) 718-7033 Fax: (701) 328-5101 *http://
www.sunflowernsa.com*

NUTRITION EDUCATION FOR THE PUBLIC (NEP)
Dietetic Practice Group 216 West Jackson Boulevard Chicago, IL
60606-6995 Phone: (312) 899-0040 *http://www.dietetics.com/
nepdpg*

OVEREATERS ANONYMOUS
P.O. Box 44020 Rio Rancho, NM 87174-4020 Phone: (505) 891-
2664 Fax: (505) 891-4320 *http://www.overeatersanonymous.org* E-
mail: *overeatr@technet.nm.org*

PRODUCE FOR BETTER HEALTH FOUNDATION
5301 Limestone Road, Suite 101 Wilmington, DE 19808-
1249 Phone: (302) 235-ADAY Fax: (302) 235-5555 *http://
www.5aday.com/*

SOCIETY FOR NUTRITION EDUCATION
7150 Winton Dr., Suite 300, Indianapolis, IN 46268 Phone:
(317)328-4627, Fax: (317)280-8527 *http://www.sne.org* E-mail:
info@sne.org

SPORTS, CARDIOVASCULAR, AND WELLNESS NUTRITIONISTS (SCAN)
90 South Cascade Avenue, Suite 1230 Colorado Springs, CO 80903 Phone: (719) 475-7751 Fax: (719) 475-8748 *http://www.nutrifit.org/*

WHEAT FOODS COUNCIL
10841 South Crossroads Drive, Suite 105 Parker, CO 80138 Phone: (303) 840-8787 Fax: (303) 840-6877 *http://www.wheatfoods.org* E-mail: *wfc@wheatfoods.org*

Government Agencies Providing Nutrition Information

CENTERS FOR DISEASE CONTROL AND PREVENTION
1600 Clifton Road, N.E. Atlanta, GA 30333 Phone: (404) 639-3311; (800) 311-3435 *http://www.cdc.gov*

FOOD AND DRUG ADMINISTRATION
Press Office 200 C Street, S.W. Washington, D.C. 20204 Phone: (202) 205-4144 *http://www.fda.gov*

FDA ADVISORY COMMITTEES
Phone: (800) 741-8138, Ext. 10564 NCTR Science Advisory Committee, Ext. 12559 FDA Food Safety and Applied Nutrition Phone: (800) FDA-4010

NATIONAL HEALTH INFORMATION CENTER
P.O. Box 1133 Washington, D.C. 20013-1133 Phone: (301) 565-4167 *http://nhic-nt.health.org*

U.S. DEPARTMENT OF AGRICULTURE
14th & Independence Avenue, S.W. Washington, D.C. 20250 Phone: (202) 720-2791 *http://www.usda.gov*

U.S. DEPARTMENT OF AGRICULTURE FOOD SAFETY AND INSPECTION SERVICE INFORMATION AND LEGISLATIVE AFFAIRS
14th Street & Independence Avenue, SW Room 1175-South Washington, D.C. 20250 Phone: (202) 720-7943 Meat and Poultry Hotline: (800) 535-4555 http://www.fsis.usda.gov

U.S. DEPARTMENT OF AGRICULTURE FOOD NUTRITION AND CONSUMER SERVICES
14th Street & Independence Avenue, S.W. Room 240-E Washington, D.C. 20250 Phone: (202) 720-7711 *http://www.usda.gov/fcs/fcs.htm*

U.S. DEPARTMENT OF AGRICULTURE NATIONAL AGRICULTURAL LIBRARY FOOD AND NUTRITION CENTER
10301 Baltimore Avenue Beltsville, MD 20705-2351 Phone: (301) 504-5719 National Labeling and Nutrition Information Center, Ext. 1 Foodborne Illness Education Information Center, Ext. 2 *http://www.nal.usda.gov*

U.S. DEPARTMENT OF HEALTH AND HUMAN SERVICES (DHHS)
200 Independence Avenue, S.W. Washington, D.C. 20201 Phone: (202) 619-0257 Fax: (202) 619-3363 *http://www.hhs.gov/*

THE WORLD HEALTH ORGANIZATION
Headquarters Office in Geneva (HQ) Avenue Appia 20 1211 Geneva 27 Switzerland Phone: (+41 22) 791 21 11 Fax: (+41 22)

791 0746 Telex: 415 416 Telegraph: UNISANTE GENEVA *http: //www.who.int/*

APPENDIX B

Eating Right With The Dietary Guidelines

THE DIETARY GUIDELINES FOR AMERICANS 2000 MAKES TEN RECOMMENDATIONS WHICH HAVE BEEN PLACED IN THREE GROUPS:

Aim for Fitness
- Aim for a healthy weight
- Be physically active each day

Build a Healthy Base
- Let the pyramid guide your food choices
- Choose a variety of grains daily, especially whole grains
- Choose a variety of fruits and vegetables daily
- Keep food safe to eat

Choose Sensibly
- Choose a diet that is low in saturated fat and cholesterol and moderate in total fat
- Choose beverages and foods to moderate your intake of sugars
- Choose and prepare foods with less salt
- If you drink alcoholic beverages, do so in moderation

APPENDIX C

In-Depth Fad Diet Book Reviews

THE SOUTH BEACH DIET

BY ARTHUR AGATSTON, M.D.

Background:

Dr. Agatston is a cardiologist in Miami Beach, Fla. This is his first diet book, and it is based on his clinical observations as well as his interpretation of the weight-loss literature.

Premise:

This book is basically about restricting, or avoiding altogether, "bad" carbs—generally refined carbs or any food with a high glycemic index. Eliminate the bad carbs and you lose weight. Allegedly, weight comes off really fast in the 14-day virtually "carb-free" Phase 1. More weight loss supposedly can be achieved during a less carb-restrictive Phase 2, which lasts "until you hit your target weight." According to Dr. Agatston, Phase 3 allows dieters to maintain their ideal weight for the rest of their lives.

THE GOOD:

- Dr. Agatston advocates many fiber-rich foods, which is a good thing. The health benefits of fiber have been well established. Also, the carbohydrate restrictions during Phases 2 and 3 are not quite as severe as some other popular low-carb plans.
- Dr. Agatston criticizes low-carb diet plans, such Dr. Atkins,

that encourage virtually unlimited amounts of foods loaded with saturated fat.

THE BAD:

- Dr. Agatston claims that his patients lost "10, 20, 30, even 50 pounds" within months, and that "they kept it off, too." However, Dr. Agatston provides no evidence to substantiate this claim, and he has not published any data in peer-reviewed journals to verify the efficacy of his diet. True to fad diet formula, the book is sprinkled with anecdotal "before-and-after" stories. Real evidence, of course, lies in the after weigh-ins. But not a single one is provided.

- The extreme weight loss promised during the 14-day induction period—8 to 13 pounds—is mostly water. The doctor's recommendation for the complete elimination of bread, rice, pasta, potatoes, all baked goods, and fruit during Phase 1 is nutritionally unsound.

- Dr. Agatston claims, "It is my purpose to teach neither low fat nor low carb. I want you to learn to choose the right fats and the right carbs." In fact, his plan is low-carb. Even in the less-restrictive Phases 2 and 3, only 20 to 30 percent of total calories come from carbohydrates. This is well below recommendations by all health organizations. A 2002 report from the National Academy of Sciences' Institute of Medicine recommended that children and adults "should consume 45 to 65 percent of their total calories from carbohydrates."

- Dr. Agatston does not think much of enriched grains: "If the label on the bread boasts that it's 'enriched,' you are really in trouble." There is no reason to believe enriched-grain products are unhealthy. While it is important to add whole-grain products to the diet because of their many health benefits, enriched-grain foods have many health benefits, too. Enrichment of grains with iron and B vitamins, for example, has helped eliminate many diseases caused by nutritional deficiencies. Folic acid enrichment alone has coincided with significantly reduced incidence of neural tube birth defects, strokes, and heart disease. It is absurd to think that "you are really in trouble" if you eat anything that is enriched.

- Although Dr. Agatston seems to favor exercise, he claims that *The South Beach Diet* "does not depend on exercise in order to work." Research shows that exercise is one of the best predictors of long-term weight maintenance. Telling an already very sedentary population that exercise is not necessary to reach and maintain an ideal weight is not good medicine.

- Even without exercise, the reader may have trouble reaching and maintaining an ideal weight. That is because beyond the initial 14-day rapid weight loss phase, the reader does not get much advice at all. Astonishingly, Dr. Agatston devotes only a half-page—less than 230 words—to describe Phase 2 (reaching ideal weight), and a similarly short-worded paragraph to describe Phase 3 (maintaining ideal weight). In fact, the book is mainly recipes.

THE UGLY:

- Carbohydrates are rated as "good" or "bad" entirely on the basis of their glycemic index (GI). By Dr. Agatston's reasoning, a peach with All-Bran (low-GI "good" carbs) makes you slim, a banana with Cheerios (high-GI "bad" carbs) makes you fat. To rate foods solely on the basis of this one criterion is overly simplistic. Strict avoidance of high-GI foods is not justified. Furthermore, the GIs of many foods listed on Dr. Agatston's GI chart differ from those listed in the 2002 International Table of Glycemic Index and Glycemic Load Values. Finally, the very premise that high-GI diets make you fat is not supported by the scientific evidence. In fact, at least two large-scale population studies fail to indicate a connection between high-GI diets and higher body weights.

- Dr. Agatston blames Americans' weight problems on the USDA Food Guide Pyramid: "National guidelines that were created to make us thin and healthy actually made us fatter and sicker." This is complete nonsense. Research shows that people who do follow the USDA Food Guide Pyramid actually *are* thinner and healthier than those who do not. It is too bad that less than 10 percent of Americans actually do follow the pyramid's guidelines. If more did, books like *The South Beach Diet* would have far fewer readers.

- Dr. Agatston claims that high-carbohydrate diets can worsen cholesterol in certain persons. Actually, most carefully controlled studies indicate that high-carbohydrate diets *reduce* cholesterol levels.

- Dr. Agatston claims that refined carbs are a recipe for weight gain and health problems, such as diabetes. To the contrary, several studies show that intake of refined carbs is associated with *lower* body weights, and does not increase risk of diabetes. Even in long-term studies that show greater weight gain associated with high consumption of refined grains as compared to whole grains, the magnitude of the difference is small (e.g., only a couple of pounds over 10 or so years). While increased consumption of whole-grain foods is a good thing, elimination of refined carbs from the diet is unnecessary—and that includes sugar. The 2002 Institute of Medicine report, mentioned above, suggests that a healthy diet can include as much as 25 percent of total calories as added sugars. In fact, most studies show that, if anything, high sugar consumption is associated with lower body weights and reduced risk of obesity!

- The book contains many bizarre and nutritionally incorrect statements. For example, Dr. Agatston asserts that "a baked potato will be less fattening with a dollop of low-fat cheese or sour cream." This is wishful thinking. Adding calories—in this case in the form of cheese or sour cream—to a fixed amount of calories (the baked potato) will be MORE fattening, not less fattening. "Even french fries are better" than a baked potato, Dr. Agatston claims, "because of the fat in which they are cooked." In other words, to lose weight, just add fat to carbs?! Again, nutritional mumbo-jumbo.

THE ULTIMATE WEIGHT SOLUTION: THE SEVEN KEYS TO WEIGHT LOSS FREEDOM

BY PHIL MCGRAW, PH.D.

Background:

Phil McGraw, Ph.D., a talk-show host and author of several self-help books.

Premise:

Getting thin depends on seven keys to "weight-loss freedom." These include (1) Right thinking (unlocks the door to self-control); (2) Healing feelings (unlocks the door to emotional control); (3) A no-fail environment (unlocks the door to external control); (4) Mastery over food and impulse eating (unlocks the door to habit control); (5) High-response cost, high-yield nutrition (unlocks the door to food control); (6) Intentional exercise (unlocks the door to body control); (7) Circle of support (unlocks the door to social control).

THE GOOD:

- Exercise is one of the seven keys. To his credit, Dr. Phil devotes an entire chapter—27 pages—to this vital component to health. Research has shown that regular exercise is vital for long-term weight control and for maintenance of weight loss.
- Dr. Phil advocates fiber-rich foods, which are important for health and long-term weight control.
- Of all the popular diet books currently on the market, the overall dietary advice in this book comes closest the dietary recommendations of the USDA's Food Guide Pyramid: 2 servings of fruit, 4 servings of vegetables, 3 servings of protein, 2 servings of low-fat dairy products; 1 serving of fat (emphasis on monounsaturated fats, fish, nuts, and seeds). The biggest drawback is the rather weak recommendation for foods that appear at the base of the USDA Food Guide Pyramid (only 2 to 3 servings/day of grains).
- Dr. Phil's recommendations for estimating portion sizes, and how to divide up the plate at mealtime in order to emphasize plant-based foods, is commendable.
- Dr. Phil at least mentions size diversity, acknowledging the genetic reality that bodies come in a variety of shapes.

THE BAD:

- Where is the evidence? Dr. Phil claims to have spent over 30 years working with overweight patients "to get results that last." In fact, he boasts that over one eight-year period in his career, he had a better than 80 percent success rate with people who were "100, 200, 300, or more pounds overweight." Not only did they lose excess weight, he claims, "they kept it off." Surprisingly, there is not a single weight-loss testimonial in this book that speaks to this astonishing record. Nor has Dr. Phil ever published any data to support these assertions. We also wonder about the other 22 years!

- Food choices come down to these: "high-response cost foods" vs. "low-response cost foods." Translation: "Good" foods vs. "bad" foods—mainly with regard to carbs. But the very definition of "good" foods is a turn-off: "High-response cost foods are those that require a great deal of work and effort to prepare and eat." Seriously, how much work is involved in consuming fresh fruits and fruit juices or whole grain breads and cereals, all of which are classified as "high-response cost foods"? Also, avoiding "low-response cost foods" seems to be based largely on whether they contain refined grains or sugar. These foods are what Dr. Phil refers to as "low-yield" foods: "high in calories but practically devoid of nutrition." Accordingly, pasta, nuts and seeds, canned and frozen fruit, and vegetables of any kind that happen to be canned or frozen in sauce, are just a few examples of foods "practically devoid of nutrition." This is nutritional nonsense. The "good vs. bad" dichotomy—with lots of "dos" and "don'ts"—is an overly simplistic view of nutrition choices, and is not likely to help anyone have a healthy relationship with food.

- Dr. Phil should have double-checked the logic of his food science. He claims that high-response cost, high-yield foods are "hunger suppressors." Low-response, low-yield foods, on the other hand, trigger overeating and lead to weight gain. The reason, he explains, is because low-response, low-yield foods cause a "seesaw effect in your blood sugar, driving it up, then letting it nose-dive. Low blood sugar leads to hunger and cravings." According to GI-based diets, this is precisely what high-glycemic foods are alleged to do, and it is apparent from Dr. Phil's bibliography for this chapter that he relies on the glycemic index to characterize carbs (e.g., Brand-Miller, et al., Glycemic Index and Obesity, *American Journal of Clinical Nutrition*, 76:281S–285S, 2002). The problem with Dr. Phil's logic, however, is that many of his so-called high-response, high-yield carbohydrates (e.g., Corn Bran, Corn Chex, Rice Chex, bananas, pineapple, mangoes) are high-glycemic. The utility of the glycemic index is debatable, and we do not recommend its use for general nutrition guidelines. Furthermore, the cereals and fruits just mentioned are perfectly good choices. The point here is that Dr. Phil recommends "hunger suppressing" foods that, according to the science he uses to support his assertions, may actually do the opposite!

- Where are the grains? In sharp contrast to the USDA Food Guide Pyramid, Dr. Phil recommends only 2 to 3 servings of what he calls "starches" (breads, grains, cereals, of starchy vegetables). Restricting these foods appears to be based on the current state of "carbophobia" in America, and certainly is not based on sound science. Many studies demonstrate the health and weight control benefits of whole grain foods.

- The book is a behavioral change weight-loss plan that is loaded with jargon. Readers have to grapple with terms such as "Minimal Effective Response" and "Weight Locus of Control," and determine whether this Weight Locus of Control is either "internal," "external," or by "chance." Although many of the behavioral recommendations that encompass Dr. Phil's seven keys to weight control are laudable (e.g., intentional exercise), it seems unlikely that the average reader will have the skills and resources to adopt them.

THE UGLY:

- Dr. Phil's definition of overweight is nothing short of incredible: "If you are overweight, then by definition, I know you are malnourished. It is true: obesity—just like starvation—is a disease of malnutrition." This statement is laughable, and seems in direct contradiction to Dr. Phil's affirmation that "God brought us into this world in a pleasing array of diverse shapes and sizes, and we are genetically programmed to be a certain way: tall, short, muscular, stout, or thin as a fiddle string." Malnutrition is a physiological condition characterized by failure to achieve nutrient requirements. It typically results from consuming too little food or a shortage or imbalance of vital nutrients. There is absolutely no justification for assuming that all people classified as overweight or obese by body mass index criteria have unbalanced diets or are lacking in key nutrients. Malnutrition can come in all sizes and shapes—just as healthy bodies can.

- Dr. Phil's body weight standards are sexist, and the men's guidelines appear to have been crafted so that Dr. Phil himself just squeaks into the recommended range. He claims that "many of the height-weight tables are based on oversimplified, obsolete formulas created more than 20 years ago." Nonetheless, Dr. Phil's weight standards for women are pretty much the same as the tables last released by MetLife, more than 20 years ago. Not so for men. The upper limit for men's weights stretches all the way into what the U.S. government and World Health Organization consider severely overweight. For example, Dr. Phil's weight table indicates that a man of average height— 5'10"—can weigh up to 206 pounds. That works out to a body mass index of 29.6, just shy of the 30.0 mark considered obese. At 6'4", Dr. Phil needs to weigh no more than 239 pounds (and hope he is "larger-boned") to make it into the okay range. Perhaps not coincidentally, that happens to be just about exactly what Dr. Phil weighs! He criticizes previous tables as being "too heavy for short people, and impossibly low for very tall men and women." Yet he does not explain why he adjusts previous tables upwards by 20 to 30 pounds for men, but not for women. We are surprised that Dr. Phil's female fans have not called him on this.

ENTER THE ZONE

by Barry Sears, Ph.D.

Background:

Barry Sears, Ph.D., is a biochemist and has authored follow-up, Zone-based diet books, including *Mastering the Zone*, *The Anti-Aging Zone*, and *A Week in the Zone*.

Premise:

According to Sears, the "zone" is a metabolic state where the mind is relaxed and focused, and the body is fluid and strong. To attain the "zone," Sears uses rigid quantities of food, apportioned in blocks, and at prescribed times. The book recommends 40 percent of calories come from carbohydrates, 30 percent of calories come from protein, and 30 percent of calories come from fat. The author believes that insulin causes weight gain, so people must attain the appropriate insulin "zone."

THE GOOD:
- Sears recommends drinking water, exercising, and snacking throughout the day.
- He acknowledges that fat is necessary in the diet.

THE BAD:
- Sears claims you can "lose weight permanently" with "exceptionally easy" rules in the "zone." In truth, complicated rules govern

every aspect of eating. Readers must calculate protein requirements based upon several tables and complex charts. They then must follow his "macronutrient block method" for determining when and how many "blocks" to eat each day. Sears further complicates the "rules" by adding another: "Never go more than five hours without eating a zone-favorable snack." Maintaining these and other rules permanently is unlikely even for the most dedicated and loyal follower.

- Sears takes the pleasure out of eating by regarding food as a medical prescription. "You must treat food as if it were a drug. You must eat food in a controlled fashion in the proper proportions—as if it were an intravenous drip." This method means EXACTLY 40 percent of calories from carbohydrates, 30 percent from fat, and 30 percent from protein at every single meal and snack. In the high-paced lifestyle of the 21st century, the last thing Americans need to follow is a strict, controlled regimen, especially when eating can and should be a pleasurable experience.

- Sears claims the average person has the stored body fat of about 1,700 pancakes and can access this body fat if following "The Zone" diet. The reality is that fat is lost if more calories are expended than taken in. People are not more likely to lose fat if they eat a certain ratio of carbohydrates, fat, and protein.

THE UGLY:
- Sears claims "The Zone" can "reset your genetic code ... because genetically, mankind has not evolved to a stage at which we can consume excessive amounts of grains and breads without adverse biochemical consequences." Your genetic code is impossible to reset—your genes are your genes. Furthermore, no scientific studies exist to suggest that eating grains and breads produces "biochemical consequences."

- Sears advises readers to not focus on calories, but then says "keep the total calories at any one meal to 500 or less—100 or less for snacks." The "Life Extension" chapter says that, for the average person, a zone-favorable diet contains no more than 800 to 1,200 calories a day. According to the book, a moderately active, 5'4" woman who weighs a healthy 125 pounds and has 23 percent body fat, should eat just 775 calories a day. In fact, any diet that recommends consuming such a low caloric intake will likely cause a person to lose weight, provided the individual can adhere to such strict guidelines. Some menus on Sears' diet call for fewer than 800 calories per day. This low-calorie recommendation may be dangerous and should be medically supervised.

- Although Sears refers throughout *Enter the Zone* to studies he has conducted to prove his diet works, not a single study is published. Even Sears' own bibliography, which readers can order by calling the 800 number at the back of the book, does not list them.

- Sears claims the insulin released as a result of eating carbohydrates causes the body to make "bad" eicosanoids (Eye-KOH-sah-noids), a substance involved in a wide range of conditions, including heart disease, cancer, arthritis, lupus, multiple sclerosis, eczema, alcoholic cravings, dull hair, dry skin, and brittle nails. This is an oversimplification of a complex process. Eicosanoids are just one part of a complex system. Although diet does somewhat affect eicosanoid levels, the effect depends primarily on what types of fatty acids one consumes—not the carbohydrate to protein ratio. The eicosanoid claim is Sears' method of capitalizing on an unfounded idea. There are no studies to suggest they are dangerous in any way.

• Sears labels certain carbohydrates as "unfavorable"—among them pasta, bananas, breakfast cereals, potatoes, breads, sandwiches, and carrots. "Unfavorable" carbohydrates are said to raise insulin levels too high, allegedly taking you out of the "zone" and into a "carbohydrate hell" that promotes obesity and other health problems. Regardless of their source, excess calories can cause weight gain. There is no scientific evidence that carbohydrates stimulate appetite and lead to more fat storage and weight gain. Contrary to this "carbohydrate hell" belief, the health benefits of complex carbohydrates are well-documented and supported by the health community. Grain foods provide numerous vitamins and minerals and are typically low fat. Because the only form of energy the brain can use is glucose (a component of complex carbohydrates), carbohydrates are of prime importance to all of us.

PROTEIN POWER

BY MICHAEL R. EADES, M.D., AND MARY DAN EADES, M.D.

Background:

Michael R. Eades, M.D., and Mary Dan Eades, M.D., are a husband and wife medical team.

Premise:

If you cut carbohydrates to "make room" for extra protein and fat, your body will be tricked into burning fat without making you feel hungry. Food should be used to condition your body, and fat is a high-octane energy source.

THE GOOD:

• The Eades recommend exercising and drinking a lot of water.

THE BAD:

- You will need to design the meals you eat based upon lists of specific foods that vary depending on whether you are in the "Intervention," "Transition," or "Maintenance" (three tiers of carbohydrate restriction) level of the program, and whether you opt for the "Hedonist," "Dilettante," or "Purist" approach (a progressive elimination of certain foods or groups of foods). Maintaining these rules permanently may be hard to do even for the most dedicated and loyal follower. With a fast-paced lifestyle, the last thing you may want to do is follow a strict, controlled eating regimen—especially when eating can and should be a pleasurable experience.

- The Eades note the earliest diet book to sweep the nation was William Banting's *Letter on Corpulence*, printed in the mid-1800s. According to the authors, "... the restricted-carbohydrate diet worked like a charm for Banting, and if sales were any indication, many others ...." Diet book sales do not necessarily indicate success. Americans spend $33 billion a year on weight-reduction programs and products, but most do not work long term. The lure of quick, easy weight loss is hard to resist, especially for those unwilling to make a commitment to lifelong behavioral change. The result? Wasted money, weight regained, a feeling of failure, and perhaps damage to health.

- The Eades claim the success of restricted-carbohydrate diets is demonstrated by the sales and popularity of books including the *Quick Weight Loss Diet* (1967), *Dr. Atkins' Diet Revolution* (1972), and *The Complete Scarsdale Medical Diet* (1979). These books in hardcover and paperback have sold over 20 million copies. "Why are they so popular? Because they work." No scientific, peer-reviewed journal has ever published any article verifying the success of any of these diets—including *Protein*

Power. At any one time in the United States, more than one-third of adult women and one-fourth of adult men are on a diet of some kind. If diets are successful, Americans would be a lean, healthy population.

- The Eades mislead readers by saying, "You would be surprised to learn that we have treated many people who have gained weight on a low-fat diet." Successful low-fat diets limit total calories. If people eat all the low-fat food they want (actually increasing the total amount of calories they consume) their weight gain would be no surprise.

THE UGLY:

- The Eades claim, "All we can tell you is that, in the almost 10 years we have been treating patients with this program, we have never had a negative outcome." In reality, no case studies of their patients with immediate results, or two- to five-year follow-ups, have been published in a scientific journal (or in their own book).

- The Eades purport that, "The actual amount of carbohydrates required by humans for health is zero." In truth, the health benefits of complex carbohydrates are well-documented and supported by the health community. Grain foods such as bread, bagels, tortillas, cereals, and pastas are typically low in fat and include essential vitamins and minerals. Because glucose is the only form of energy the brain can use, carbohydrates are of prime importance to all of us.

- The authors define eicosanoids as "... a gang of at least 100 powerful hormone-like substances that control virtually all physiological action in your body." However, eicosanoids are one part of a complex system. According to Ellen Coleman, M.A., R.D., M.P.H., "The belief that eicosanoids control all physiological functions (including athletic performance, health, and disease) is not only unfounded, it is an appalling over-simplification of complex physiological processes." (*Source: Int. J. Sports Nutr.*, 6: 69–71, 1996.)

DR. BOB ARNOT'S REVOLUTIONARY WEIGHT CONTROL PROGRAM

BY ROBERT ARNOT, M.D.

Background:
Robert Arnot, M.D., is the chief medical correspondent for NBC News and appears regularly on "CBS Evening News" and "Dateline." He also writes a monthly column for *Self* magazine.

Premise:
Foods are drugs. Eating certain foods will make you feel terrible and gain weight, while other foods will guarantee weight loss. The book proposes to alter the body's physiology from weight gain to weight loss. Arnot promotes consuming "hard foods"—ones with high soluble fiber—and a "feedforward" eating plan—which will teach you in what order and at what times of day to eat foods to maximally control your weight, hunger, and mood.

THE GOOD:
- Dr. Arnot promotes eating fiber as a healthful weight-loss tool.

THE BAD:
- Arnot says his friends suggest, "I am not a weight-loss specialist but I play one on TV." If he is not a weight-loss specialist, then Arnot should not have written a diet book.

- Arnot claims one of the greatest weight-loss benefits of protein is that it is "brain energizing." In reality, glucose is the only form of energy the brain can use; its primary source in the diet is carbohydrates, not protein.

- You will need to design the meals you eat based upon "Feedforward Eating," which will teach you in what order and at what times of day to eat to maximally control your weight. The day is divided into zones (The Power Zone, The Loading Zone, The Craving Zone, The Relaxation Zone, The Fat Zone, and The Workout Zone), each of which is complete with its own meal plan. For each zone, there are multiple meals from which you can pick and choose. You may have a hard time maintaining these rules permanently, even if you're a dedicated and loyal follower. With a fast-paced lifestyle, the last thing you may want to do is follow a strict, controlled eating regimen—especially when eating can and should be a pleasurable experience.

- Arnot claims that "Foods with a high-glycemic index, from instant mashed potatoes and white breads, Twinkies and muffins, to bagels, are digested very quickly, giving rise to high blood sugars and placing a heavy 'load' on your body. Since these high-glucose foods are basically glucose bombs, the more of these foods in your diet, the higher your 'glucose load.'" Carbohydrates are rarely eaten individually—they are usually eaten in combination with protein, fat, and other low glycemic index foods that moderate any spikes in blood sugar. Additionally, basing a person's diet purely on a food's glycemic index further adds to the confusion. Potatoes, white bread, bagels, pasta, and muffins all provide essential vitamins and minerals and are typically low in fat. Avoiding these nutritious foods because of their glycemic index means a person may miss out on valuable nutrients.

THE UGLY:

- Although Arnot claims, "The ideas in this book aren't just theoretical science. They have worked for hundreds of people who have had an early look at perfect weight control …"—his premise is unfounded. Scientifically validated studies are the cornerstones for basic nutrition principles, not anecdotes from friends and relatives. Arnot's "validation" for his book comes from "… people who have had an early look at perfect weight control, from my editor at Little, Brown, my producers at work, scientific colleagues, 100,000 readers of *Turning Back the Clock*, to my wife, children, and friends."

- Arnot predicts that, "Ten years from now, you will be able to manipulate your appetite and weight easily with genetically engineered drugs based on newly discovered hormones …." With Fen-Phen diet drugs being yanked from market shelves in September 1997 because of potentially deadly side effects, and the past failure from the 1960s amphetamine diet pills, there is evidence that weight-loss drugs probably will never be the magic bullet that many consumers hope.

- "Refined carbohydrates such as those in white flour breads, bagels, muffins, and snack foods … can cause such rapid gains in weight. These foods are the dietary equivalent of 'crack,' since you would have to hammer yourself all day long with them to keep feeling good," claims Arnot. In fact, there is no scientific evidence that carbohydrates stimulate appetite and lead to more fat storage and weight gain. Weight gain occurs when intake is greater than output, regardless of food type. Anyone can gain weight from eating all types of food, provided we eat more than we expend.

- Arnot claims a diet high in protein and low in carbohydrates will decrease your hunger and, therefore, lead to weight loss.

This claim runs counter to healthful eating guidelines recommended by the Food Guide Pyramid. Food intake study reports, such as the U.S. Department of Agriculture's (USDA) Healthy Eating Index, show Americans already eat plenty of protein and fat, but fall short of meeting dietary goals for grain, fruits, and vegetables. Additional studies also agree with the USDA findings: most Americans do not get enough complex carbohydrates from grain foods such as breads, cereals, pastas, barley, and rice.

THE CARBOHYDRATE ADDICT'S LIFESPAN PROGRAM: A PERSONALIZED PLAN FOR BECOMING SLIM, FIT, AND HEALTHY IN YOUR 40s, 50s, 60s, AND BEYOND

BY RICHARD F. HELLER, M.S., PH.D., AND RACHAEL F. HELLER, M.A., M.PH., PH.D.

Background:

Richard F. Heller, M.S., Ph.D., and Rachael F. Heller, M.A., M.Ph., Ph.D., are a husband-wife team—he is a biologist, she is a psychologist.

Premise:

An excess of insulin, the "hunger hormone," causes the carbohydrate addict to experience intense and recurring cravings, as well as the heightened ability to store fat. The authors stress that the affected person has a biological condition caused by a hormonal imbalance, and that the imbalance can be corrected by following their "STAR program"—Simple, Targeted to one's needs and decade of life, Adaptable to one's lifestyle, and Rewards a person with food they love." The first step is the "basic plan": eating a balanced "Reward Meal" every day, completing the "Reward Meal" within one hour, and eating only craving-reducing foods at all other meals and snacks. After two weeks, begin to add "options" if necessary (one at a time).

THE GOOD:

- The Hellers condemn prejudice toward people who are overweight. They also realize that some carbohydrate-rich foods are needed for "energy, nutrition, and satisfaction" and allow all foods to be included in the diet somewhere. They stress the importance of choosing a realistic weight goal based on your age, body build, and health needs, and recommend a reasonable weight loss of one-half to two pounds a week.

THE BAD:

- The Hellers claim that you can lose weight and keep it off with simple guidelines and "no calorie counting, no measuring, and no food exchanges." Although the Hellers have refined their initial recommendations into only three guidelines, there are a lot of options, meal plans, and even more recipes (more than 200). Maintaining these and other rules permanently is unlikely even for the most dedicated follower. It is ironic that the Hellers claim, "You will be able to make lifestyle changes virtually without effort." The Hellers take the pleasure out of eating by treating food like a medical prescription—"make sure to maintain 1/3, 1/3, 1/3 portions at the Reward Meal."
- The Hellers proclaim, "big business appears to play a major role in the low-fat, cure-all push." There is no such thing as a "cure-all" way of eating that automatically protects you from disease. A low-fat diet may still fall short if it is high in calories or lacking in variety. Ironically, the Hellers seem to be contributing significantly to the $33 billion "big business" weight-loss industry, as the *Carbohydrate Addict's Life Span Program* retails

for $15.95, and their other six books retail at a total of $81.83.

- Exercise is not discussed in the Hellers' program except as an option that can be added, if necessary, to further reduce insulin and cravings. The American Heart Association, the American Dietetic Association, and the American Medical Association all agree, the most sensible approach to weight loss is a balanced diet combined with exercise. Engaging in mild or moderate activity greatly helps a person lose/maintain their weight, which may, in turn, decrease blood fats. A person who exercises also will reap health benefits—increased "good" cholesterol, a maintenance in lean body mass, and decreased risk of type 2 diabetes.

- Success is demonstrated by personal testimonials. Scientifically validated studies are the cornerstones for basic nutrition principles, not anecdotes from the Hellers' patients or Rachael or Richard's personal success stories. The Hellers' "validation" for their book also comes from "… our research" and "other researchers." No success-rate data or case studies of the Hellers' followers are published anywhere in their book or in a scientific journal.

- The Hellers' state "Our research indicates that up to 75 percent of the overweight, and as many as 40 percent of the normal-weight, are carbohydrate addicted. Other researchers have reported similar numbers, or varying numbers, depending on the age, gender, and ethnic differences of the people they have studied." The notion of a physiological carbohydrate "addiction" has not been supported by research. To the contrary, studies have found that sugar is not unique among carbohydrates as a dietary component affecting food intake [*Am J Clin Nutr.*, 62:195–201, 1995], and that carbohydrate intake does not increase hunger [*Physiol Behav.*, 58:421–7, 1995]. "Addiction" is not a word to be taken lightly—so if anything, the role of carbohydrates, food-related cognitions, and "cravings" should be further explored.

- The program dictates you must weigh yourself each day and record your weight on the Progress Chart in order to calculate your weekly average weight loss (and the weekly weight loss you can probably expect in the weeks to come). Throw out the scale. For some women, weight can fluctuate from three to five pounds on a daily basis, and the weights of men will naturally vary by several pounds as well. Having people pay too much attention to their weight, rather than healthy eating habits, may set them up for disappointment.

THE UGLY:
- The authors believe carbohydrates cause blood sugar levels to rise and crank up insulin production, which promotes fat storage. In reality, the body does produce insulin in response to rises in blood sugar, but insulin promotes fat storage only when a person consumes excess calories. The authors' view of insulin is overly simplistic. In truth, insulin is an essential hormone that helps transfer the natural sugars of digested foods from the bloodstream to the body's cells, where these sugars fuel our activities.
- There is no scientific basis for the Hellers' insulin weight-loss theory, or evidence to suggest that carbohydrates stimulate appetite and lead to more fat storage and weight gain. Many experts argue that obesity leads to excessive insulin production, independent of carbohydrate consumption. There is no scientific evidence that carbohydrates stimulate appetite or lead to fat storage and weight gain. Furthermore, the health benefits of complex carbohydrates are well-documented and well-supported by the health community.

- The Hellers pay lip service to "cutting" fat in the diet at the very end of the book. Fat actually accounts for 45 to 70 percent of total calories on the Hellers' diet—well above the 30 percent limit recommended by most health professionals. Even with small portions and omitting second helpings and snacks, the daily intake for three sample menus averaged almost 2000 calories. Most women need this amount to maintain their weight, not lose it.

- The Hellers believe breakfast is not essential for health or weight loss/maintenance. They claim, "You can choose to skip breakfast or have only a cup of coffee or tea." Breakfast is essential. It gives us a substantial part of the day's recommended nutrients. Data from the U.S. Department of Agriculture shows that cognitive abilities may be enhanced by breakfast, perhaps optimally with sufficient carbohydrates to elevate glucose for several hours. Research also shows people who select ready-to-eat cereals for breakfast eat fewer calories from fat over the entire day, get more fiber in their diet, and consume 20 percent more of essential vitamins and minerals than on non-cereal days.

- Although the Hellers tout the benefits of fiber by saying "… a low-fat diet without high fiber is worthless in terms of decreasing blood fat," they never once mention fiber as playing a key role in weight loss. Based upon their menu recommendations, it is highly unlikely that the Hellers' diet would allow anyone to consume the recommended 20 to 35 grams of fiber per day. By and large, a diet that is lower in fat will be naturally higher in fiber—neither of which are the case for the Hellers' diet. A high intake of dietary fiber may be an effective means of reducing obesity, high blood pressure, and other heart disease risk factors, according to a cohort study published in the recent October 27 issue of the *Journal of the American Medical Association*. In addition to fiber's protective effect against certain types of cancers and gastrointestinal disorders, some studies have found a high-fiber meal is satiating, decreases the length of a meal and may decrease intake at the next meal.

- The sad truth is, not only would someone following the Hellers' diet be missing out on fiber, they also would be depriving themselves of the phytochemicals, vitamins, and minerals that may help prevent cancer and heart disease.

DR. ATKINS' NEW DIET REVOLUTION

BY ROBERT C. ATKINS, M.D.

Background:

A Cornell Medical School graduate, Dr. Robert Atkins was a practicing physician for over 30 years, and was the founder and medical director of the Atkins' Center for Complementary Medicine in New York City. A self-proclaimed leader in the natural medicine and nutritional pharmacology areas, Dr. Atkins authored a string of weight-loss books, since his original book, *Dr. Atkins' Diet Revolution*, was published in 1972. In addition, Atkins manufactures several low-carbohydrate food products trademarked under the Atkins Diet brand name, as well as a line of "Vita Nutrient" solutions.

Premise:

Atkins' premise hinges on one basic factor in the control of obesity—excessive amounts of insulin govern the basic mechanism by which the body lays on fat. The diet promises you can still lose pounds and inches while you eat as many, or even more, calories than you might normally, from predominantly protein and fat-laden foods. The one requirement is that you must drastically reduce your intake of dietary carbohydrates, thus forcing the body to burn your reserve of stored fat for energy.

THE GOOD:

- Dr. Atkins admits that, in addition to his diet, dieters may need to add another leg to the program—exercise. He devotes a full chapter of his book to the benefits of exercise, noting that, if weight loss is to be successful, increasing physical activity is a must.

- Atkins suggests everyone have a medical checkup to determine general health status prior to embarking on the diet.

THE BAD:

- The diet promotes one food element over another—it is unbalanced and excessively high in protein and fat. Typical of many high-protein weight-loss regimes, Atkins' diet provides limited food choices, primarily limiting carbohydrates. Atkins states, however, that on his diet, you may eat less fat overall from increased meat, fish, fowl, eggs, and butter consumption. It is highly unlikely the diet would contain low levels of fat, given the fact that unlimited consumption of meat, eggs, and cheese is recommended—even in the first stage of his diet, called the "Induction" stage. A diet rich in fat and cholesterol—especially saturated fat—can increase the risk of developing cardiovascular disease and some cancers.

- Atkins claims sugar and refined carbohydrates are bad for your health, bad for your energy level, bad for your mental state, bad for your figure, bad for your career prospects, bad for your sex life, bad for your digestion, bad for your blood chemistry, and bad for your heart. No food is bad for your health when eaten in moderation. All foods can fit into a healthy diet. In reality, carbohydrates provide essential calories for children at times of growth and development. Furthermore, a report issued by the Food and Agriculture Organization (FAO) and the World Health Organization (WHO) confirmed the importance of carbohydrates in the diet, noting carbohydrates can help reduce the risk of obesity and protect against certain cancers. The report also stated no evidence exists that indicates sugars and starches promote obesity.

- Patients have taught Atkins that 90 percent of the time, being overweight was caused by a disturbed carbohydrate metabolism. He further states that the high carbohydrate, 30 percent fat diet is "mythology based on some well-observed scientific facts poorly interpreted," and has caused the American obesity epidemic. Atkins states the American public has been brainwashed into thinking the high-carbohydrate diet is the only proper and healthy diet for a human being. The Atkins' diet advises eating fewer carbohydrates and more protein than is recommended in the Food Guide Pyramid and the U.S. Dietary Guidelines, which are based on scientific evidence and advocated by healthcare professionals nationwide. Research has shown high saturated fat diets, such as those Atkins promotes, are detrimental to health and more likely to cause obesity.

- Atkins indicates not being hungry is a typical result of being in Benign Dietary Ketoacidosis (BDK). Atkins claims BDK will eventually lead to decreased hunger and give the dieter a metabolic advantage. A diet full of "metabolic advantages" allows you to "sneak them (calories) out of your body, unused or dissipated, as heat." You do not "sneak" calories out. Fat is lost only when more calories are expended than ingested. Furthermore, food intake reports, such as the U.S. Department of Agriculture's (USDA) Healthy Eating Index, show Americans already eat plenty of protein and fat, but fall short of meeting dietary goals for grain, fruits, and vegetables. At the same time, studies show Americans are heavier than they were 20 years ago.

- Dr. Atkins claims weight loss on his diet is very fast and significant, "the diet is so effective at dissolving adipose tissue that it can create fat loss greater than occurs in fasting." Successful and safe weight loss does not happen overnight or even in a week or two. It requires a great deal of effort and a commitment to healthy lifestyle changes. "If you want to lose weight, you must restrict calories" says Dr. Margo Denke, associate professor of internal medicine at the Center for Human Nutrition, Southwestern Medical Center, Dallas.

- What Atkins fails to point out is, the real reason people are losing weight is that they are simply eating fewer calories.

- Dr. Atkins advocates "supplements for everyone"—a broad multivitamin, L-glutamine for sugar cravers, borage oil, lecithin granules, and pantethine. Just as losing weight does not happen overnight, there is no "magic" pill that will eliminate unwanted pounds. Moreover, consumers should rely on whole foods, rather than pills, to provide essential minerals and nutrients.

THE UGLY:

- Without carbohydrates, the body does not burn fat efficiently, and substances called ketones accumulate in the blood. Atkins states that this condition, "ketosis," is not only pleasurable, but frequently essential—the "key" to excising obesity with the precision of a skilled surgeon, who dissects away a tumor while leaving the healthy tissue intact. The release of ketones—evident in the breath and in the urine—is a good thing to experience, he says, because it is proof positive the body is consuming stored fat. Ketosis may make dieting seem easier (at least initially) due to rapid water loss and a reduced appetite. However, this condition is often accompanied by nausea, headaches, fatigue, and bad breath—side effects most people would find undesirable.

- Atkins suggests prolonged fasting can be dangerous and has one severe metabolic disadvantage—the catabolism of lean muscle tissue. He claims, however, investigation has shown that, on his diet, virtually no lean tissue is lost, only adipose tissue. High-protein diets make it more difficult for the body to absorb minerals such as calcium and may put you at greater risk of developing osteoporosis. This diet not only shortchanges the body by excluding proper amounts of other nutrients but, over time, it also may place excessive demands on the kidneys and liver. It potentially can lead to dehydration because more fluid is required to rid the body of nitrogen if protein is used mostly for energy. In some cases, existing medical conditions, such as kidney disease and gout, can be exacerbated.

- Atkins admits the body powers its operations mainly through the use of glucose in the blood—it must have glucose. But he goes on to say it does not need to come from one's diet. His solution is ketosis and lipolysis—which is "the process of dissolving fat." Glucose is the primary form of energy the brain can use, and the primary source for glucose in the diet is carbohydrate, not protein. The body has to break down lean body tissue to convert protein to carbohydrates to fuel the brain. In the process, you lose lean tissue, lots of water, and weight.

SUGAR BUSTERS!

BY H. LEIGHTON STEWARD, MORRISON C. BETHEA, M.D., SAM S. ANDREWS, M.D., AND LUIS A. BALART, M.D.

Background:

H. Leighton Steward holds a geology degree and is the CEO of an energy company; Morrison C. Bethea, M.D., is a cardiologist; Sam S. Andrews, M.D., is an endocrinologist; and Luis A. Balart, M.D., is a gastroenterologist.

Premise:

Eating sugar causes the body to release insulin, a hormone that promotes fat storage, and obesity results from this insulin overload. *Sugar Busters!* advises against carbohydrates—especially refined and processed ones. According to the authors, decreasing sugar intake can help you trim body fat and lose weight, regardless of whatever else you eat.

THE GOOD:

- Whole grains and some vegetables are allowed on the *Sugar Busters!* plan.

THE BAD:

- The authors state, "We would like to write a thick, fine-print book about all this good news, but a book that covers the weight-loss implications of this way of eating has already been written by Michel Montignac of France, and William Dufty has described the evil effects of sugar itself in his *Sugar Blues*." A book that bases its diet premises upon obscure books published in 1976 and 1991 by unknown authors without health backgrounds should raise suspicions about *Sugar Busters!* claims and recommendations. What's more, the authors' list contains only 20 references throughout the book, many of them unknown textbooks and journals.

- According to the authors, "You must virtually eliminate potatoes, corn, white rice, bread from refined flour, beets, carrots and, of course, refined sugar, corn syrup, molasses, honey, sugared colas, and beer. Beyond that, you should eat fruit by itself. The list of foods allowed on the diet is extensive and will delight you by its length and variety." An enduring motto of the American Dietetic Association reminds consumers that "All Foods Can Fit." In fact, the authors' suggestions to limit specific grain foods and fruits and vegetables run counter to the Food Guide Pyramid recommendations. Food intake study reports such as the USDA's Healthy Eating Index show Americans already eat plenty of protein and fat, but fall short of meeting dietary goals for grains, fruits, and vegetables. This advice ignores the nutritional value, vitamins, and minerals these foods contribute to the diet.

THE UGLY:

- The authors claim, "Let's get to the point. SUGAR IS TOXIC! Sugar? Some sugar? Most sugar? All sugar? Toxic? Well, we will say refined sugar in any significant quantity is toxic to many human bodies, and it certainly helps to make many bodies fat." A joint report released April 5, 1998, by the Food and Agriculture Organization (FAO) and the World Health Organization (WHO) confirmed the importance of carbohydrates in the diet, noting that a high-carbohydrate intake can reduce the risk of obesity and protect against nutrition-related diseases. Another key finding of the report showed no evidence exists that sugars and starches promote obesity. Excess food consumption in any form, on the other hand, will promote body-fat accumulation if intake is not matched by energy expenditure. The authors themselves admit they don't exercise.

- The authors recommend that, "In general, fluids should be drunk in small quantities during meals. 'Washing' food down frequently causes the bypass of proper chewing which is necessary to break food into smaller, more appropriate particles for better digestion. Excess fluid with meals also dilutes the digestive juices … which may result in partially digested food." No scientific evidence exists to support the claim that consuming fluids during a meal negatively affects digestion. What's more, health professionals stress the importance of consuming fluids for maintaining and regulating fluid balance, preventing headaches and fatigue associated with dehydration, and helping with weight loss. A sedentary individual needs at least eight glasses of fluid each day, and an active individual needs at least 10.

- The authors believe carbohydrates cause the blood sugar to rise and crank up insulin production, which promotes fat storage. The author's view of insulin's role is overly simplistic. In reality, the body produces insulin in response to rises in blood sugar, but insulin promotes fat storage only when a person consumes excess calories. There is no scientific basis for the *Sugar Busters!* insulin weight-loss theory. Many experts argue that obesity leads to excessive insulin production, independent of carbohydrate consumption.

- The authors demonstrate questionable research methods, stating, "With our approach, many individuals already have experienced significant weight loss and reduction in cholesterol (an average of approximately 15 percent) as well as improvement in performance, which is so vital to everyone's success. In addition, many diabetics have been successful in achieving much better regulation of their blood sugar levels." No success-rate data or case studies of their followers are published anywhere in their book or in a scientific journal. If a reader calls the phone number at the back of the book, he or she must leave a message.

REFERENCES

CHAPTER 1

Anderson, J. W., Konz, E. C., and Jenkins, D. J. A. "Health advantages and disadvantages of weight-reducing diets: A computer analysis and critical review." Journal of the American College of Nutrition, 19: 578-590, 2000.

Barnard, R.J., "Effects of life-style modification on serum lipids," Archives of Internal Medicine, Vol. 151, No. 1, p. 389-1 394, 1991.

Blundell, J.E., and Burley, V.J., "Evaluation of the satiating power of dietary fat in man," Progress in Obesity Research (Y. Oomura et al., eds.), John Libbey & Company Ltd., p. 453-457, 1990.

Bravata, D. M., Sanders, L., Huang, J., Krumholz, H. M., Olkin, I., Gardner, C. D., Bravata, D., M. "Efficacy and safety of low-carbohydrate diets: A systematic review." Journal of the American Medical Association, 289: 1837-1850, 2003.

Bowman, S. A., and Spence, J. T. "A comparison of low-carbohydrate vs. high-carbohydrate diets: Energy restriction, nutrient quality and correlation to body mass index." Journal of the American College of Nutrition, 21: 268-274, 2002.

Danforth, E., "Dietary obesity," American Journal of Clinical Nutrition, 41:1132-1145, 1985.

Denke, M. A. "Metabolic effects of high-protein, low-carbohydrate diets." The American Journal of Cardiology, 88: 59-61, 2001.

Fleming, R. M. "The effect of high-, moderate-, and low-fat diets on weight loss and cardiovascular disease risk factors." Preventive Cardiology, 5: 110-118, 2002.

Foster-Powell, K., Holt, S. H. A., and Brand-Miller, J. C. "International table of glycemic index and glycemic load values: 2002." American Journal of Clinical Nutrition, 76: 5-56, 2002.

Fukagawa, N.K., Anderson, J.W., Hageman, G., Young, V.R., Minaker, K.L., "High-carbohydrate, high-fiber diets increase peripheral insulin sensitivity in healthy young and old adults," American Journal of Clinical Nutrition, 52:5240-528, 1990.

Gaesser, G.A., Big Fat Lies: The Truth About Your Weight and Your Health, Fawcett Columbine, New York, 1996.

Hays, N. P., Starling R.D., Liu, X., Sullivan, D. H., Trappe, T. A., Fluckey, J. D., Evans, W. D. "Effects of an ad libitum low-fat, high-carbohydrate diet on body weight, body composition, and fat distribution in older men and women." Archives of Internal Medicine, 164: 210-217, 2004.

Jequier, E., "Body weight regulation in humans: the importance of nutrient balance," News in Physiological Sciences, 8: 273-276, 1993.

Jequier, E., and Bray, G. A. "Low-fat diets are preferred." American Journal of Medicine, 113(9B): 41S-46#, 2002.

Kendall, A., Levitsky, D.A., Strupp, B.J., and Lissner, L., "Weight loss on a low-fat diet: Consequence of the imprecision of the control of food intake in humans," American Journal of Clinical Nutrition, 53: 1124-1129, 1991.

Kennedy, E.T., Bowman, S. A., Spence, J. T., Freedman, M., King, J. "Popular diets: Correlation to health, nutrition, and obesity." Journal of the American Dietetic Association, 101: 411-420, 2001.

Keys, A., Brozek, J., Henschel, A., Michelson, O., and Taylor, H.L., Biology of Human Starvation, Univ. Minn. Press, Minnesota, 1950.

Kuczmarski, R.J., Flegal, K.M., Campbell, S.M., and Johnson, C.L., "Increasing prevalence of overweight among U.S. adults," The National Health and Nutrition Examination Surveys, 1960 to 1961, Journal of the American Medical Association, 272:205-211, 1994.

Larosa, J.C., Fry, A.G., Muesing, R., and Rosing, D.R., "Effects of high-protein, low-carbohydrate dieting on plasma lipoproteins and body weight," Journal of the American Dietetic Association, 77:264–270, 1980.

Leibel, R.L., Rosenbaum, M., and Hirsch, J., "Changes in energy expenditure resulting from altered body weight," New England Journal of Medicine, 332:621-628, 1995.

Lovejoy, J., and DiGirolamo, M., "Habitual dietary intake and insulin sensitivity in lean and obese adults," American Journal of Clinical Nutrition, 52:1174-1179, 1992.

Ludwig, D.S., Pereira, M.A., and Kroenke, C.H., "Dietary Fiber, Weight Gain, and Cardiovascular Disease Risk Factors in Young Adults," Journal of the American Medical Association, 282: 1539-1546, 1999.

Meyer, K. A., Kushi, L. H., Jacobs, D. R., Slavin, J., Sellers, T. A., and Folsom, A. R. "Carbohydrates, dietary fiber, and incident type 2 diabetes in older women." American Journal of Clinical Nutrition, 71: 921-930, 2000.

NIH Technology Assessment Conference Panel, "Methods for voluntary weight loss and control," Annals of Internal Medicine, 119: 764-760, 1993.

Poppitt, S. D., Keogh, G. F., and Prentice, A. M., et al. "Long-term effects of ad libitum low-fat, high-carbohydrate diets on body weight and serum lipids in overweight subjects with metabolic syndrome." American Journal of Clinical Nutrition, 75: 11-20, 2002.

Prewitt, T.E., Schmeisser, D., Bowen, P.E., Aye, P., Dolecek, T.A., Langenburg, P., Cole, T., and Brace, L, "Changes in body weight, body composition, and energy intake in women fed high- and low-fat diets," American. Journal of Clinical Nutrition, 54:304-310, 1991.

Rickman, F., Mitchell, N., Dingman, J., and Dalen, J.E., "Changes in serum cholesterol during the Stillman diet," Journal of the American Medical Association, 228:54-58, 1974.

Saris, W. H. M. "Sugars, energy metabolism, and body weight control." American Journal of Clinical Nutrition, 78 (Suppl): 850S-857S, 2003.

Shick, S.M., Wing, R.R., and Klem, K.L., et al., "Persons successful at long-term weight loss and maintenance continue to consume a low-energy, low-fat diet," Journal of the American Dietetic Association, 98:408-413, 1998.

West, K.M., Epidemiology of diabetes and its vascular lesions, Elsevier, New York, 1978.

Westman, E. C., Yancy, W. S., Edman, J. S., Tomlin, K. F., Perkins, C. E. "Effect of 6-month adherence to a very low carbohydrate diet program." American Journal of Medicine, 113: 30-36, 2002.

Wolk, A., Manson, J.E., and Stampfer, M.J., et al., "Long-term intake of dietary fiber and decreased risk of coronary heart disease among women," Journal of the American Medical Association, 281:1998-2004, 1999.

Yang, E. J., Kerver, J. M., Park, Y., K., Kayitsinga, J., Allison, D. B., and Song, W. O. "Carbohydrate intake and biomarkers of glycemic control among US adults: the third National Health and Nutrition Examination Survey (NHANES III)." American Journal of Clinical Nutrition, 77: 1426-1433, 2003.

CHAPTER 2

Duyff, Roberta L., The American Dietetic Association's Complete Food & Nutrition Guide, Chronimed Publishing, Minneapolis, 1998.

Fung, T. T., Hu, F. B., Pereira, M. A., Liu, S., Stampfer, M. J., Colditz, G. A., Willett, W. C. "Whole-grain intake and the risk of type 2 diabetes: a prospective study in men." American Journal of Clinical Nutrition, 76: 535-540, 2002.

Hu, F. B. "The mediterranean diet and mortality—olive oil and beyond." New England Journal of Medicine, 348: 2595-2596, 2003.

Kant, A., Schatzkin, A., and Graubard, B., et. al, "A Prospective Study of Diet Quality and Mortality in Women," Journal of the American Medical Association, 283:2109-2115, 2000.

Liese, A. D., Roach, A. K., Sparks, K. C., Marquart, L., D-Agostino, R. B., Mayer-Davis, E., J. "Whole-grain intake and insulin sensitivity: the Insulin Resistance Atherosclerosis Study." American Journal of Clinical Nutrition, 78: 965-971, 2003.

Liu, S., Sesso, H.D., Manson, J. E., Willett, W. C., Buring, J. E. "Is intake of breakfast cereals related to total and cause-specific mortality in men?" American Journal of Clinical Nutrition, 77: 594-599, 2003.

McKeown, N. M., Meigs, J. B., Liu, S., Wilson, P. W. F., and Jacques, P. F. "Whole-grain intake is favorably associated with metabolic risk factors for type 2 diabetes and cardiovascular disease in the Framingham Offspring Study." American Journal of Clinical Nutrition, 76: 390-398, 2002.

Merchant, A. T., Hu, F. B., Spiegelman, D., Willett, W. C., Rimm, E. B., Ascherio, A. "Dietary fiber reduces peripheral arterial disease risk in men." Journal of Nutrition, 133: 3658-3663, 2003.

Montonen, J., Knekt, P., Jarvinen, R., Aromaa, A., and Reunanen, A. "Whole-grain and fiber intake and the incidence of type 2 diabetes." American Journal of Clinical Nutrition, 77: 622-629, 2003.

Painter, J., Rah, J.-H., and Lee, Y.-K. "Comparison of international food guide pictorial representations." Journal of the American Dietetic Association,102: 483-489, 2002.

Pereira, M. A., O'Reilly, E., and Augustsson, K., et al. "Dietary fiber and risk of coronary heart disease. A pooled analysis of cohort studies." Archives of Internal Medicine, 164: 370-376, 2004.

Song, Y., Buring, J.E., Manson, J. E., and Liu, S. "Dietary magnesium intake in relation to plasma insulin levels and risk of type 2 diabetes in women." Diabetes Care, 27: 59-65, 2004.

Tribole, Evelyn, Stealth Health, Penguin Putnam, Inc., New York, 1998.

Venti, C. A., and Johnson, C. S. "Modified food guide pyramid for lactovegetarians and vegans." Journal of Nutrition, 132: 1050-1054, 2002.

Wolk, A., Manson, J. E., Stampfer, M. J., Colditz, G. A., Hu, F. B., Speizer, F. E., Hennekens, C. H., and Willett, W. C. "Long-term intake of dietary fiber and decreased risk of coronary heart disease among women." Journal of the American Medical Association, 281: 1998-2004, 1999.

Wu, H., Dwyer, K., M., Fan, Z., Shircore, A., Fan, J., Dwyer, J. H. "Dietary fiber and progression of atherosclerosis: the Los Angeles Atherosclerosis Study." American Journal of Clinical Nutrition, 78: 1085-1091, 2003.

CHAPTER 3

Duyff, Roberta L, The American Dietetic Association's Complete Food & Nutrition Guide, Chronimed Publishing, Minneapolis, 1998.

Institute of Medicine, National Academy of Sciences. "Dietary reference intakes for energy, carbohydrate, fiber, fat, fatty acids, cholesterol, protein, and amino acids." Executive Summary, September 2002.

Kant, A., Schatzkin, A., and Graubard, B., et. al, "A Prospective Study of Diet Quality and Mortality in Women," Journal of the American Medical Association, 283:2109-2115, 2000.

Linebeck, D. R., and Miller Jones, J. "Sugars and health workshop: summary and conclusions." American Journal of Clinical Nutrition, 78 (suppl): 893S-897S, 2003.

Murphy, S. P., and Johnson, R. K. "The scientific basis of recent US guidance on sugar intake." American Journal of Clinical Nutrition, 78 (Suppl): 827S-833S, 2003.

Satter, E., How To Get Your Kid To Eat … But Not Too Much, Bull Publishing Co., Palo Alto, Calif., 1987.

Tribole, Evelyn, Stealth Health, Penguin Putnam, Inc., New York, 1998.

CHAPTER 4

Harris, R.B., "Role of set-point theory in regulation of body weight," Federation of American Societies for Experimental Biology Journal, 4:3310-3318, 1990.

Keesey, R.E., and Powley, T.L., "The regulation of body weight," Annual Review of Psychology, 37:109-133, 1986.

Lee, C.D., Blair, S.N., and Jackson, A.S., "Cardiorespiratory fitness, body composition, and all-cause and cardiovascular disease mortality in men," American Journal of Clinical Nutrition, 69: 373-380, 1999.

NIH Publication, "NHLBI Guidelines on the Identification, Evaluation, and Treatment of Overweight and Obesity in Adults," The Evidence Report, No. 98-4083.

CHAPTER 5

Kratina, Karin, King, Nancy, and Hayes, Dayle, Moving Away From Diets: New Ways to Heal Eating Problems and Exercise Resistance, Helm Seminars, Publishing, Lake Dallas, Texas, 1996.

Tribole, Evelyn, and Resch, Elyse, Intuitive Eating: A Recovery Book for the Chronic Dieter, St. Martin's Press, New York, 1995.

CHAPTER 6

Ainsworth, B.E., Haskell, W.H., and Leon, A.S., et al., "Compendium of physical activities: classification of energy costs of human physical activities," Medical Science Sports Exercise, 25:71–80, 1993.

American College of Sports Medicine, "Position Stand: The recommended quantity and quality of exercise for developing and maintaining cardiorespiratory and muscular fitness, and flexibility in healthy adults," Medical Science Sports Exercise, 30: 975-991, 1998.

Kratina, Karin, King, Nancy, and Hayes, Dayle, Moving Away From Diets: New Ways to Heal Eating Problems and Exercise Resistance, Helm Seminars, Publishing, Lake Dallas, Texas, 1996.

Borg, G.A., "Psychophysical bases of perceived exertion," Medical Science Sports Exercise, Vol. 14, No. 6, p. 377-381, 1982.

Pate, R.R., et al., "Physical activity and public health. A recommendation from the Centers for Disease Control and Prevention and the American College of Sports Medicine," Journal of the American Medical Association, 273:402-407, 1995.

Peterson, J.A., and Balke, B., The Fitness Handbook, Sagmore Publishing, Inc., Champagne, Ill., 1995.

U.S. Department of Health and Human Services, "Physical Activity and Health," A report of the Surgeon General, U.S. Department of Health and Human Services, Centers for Disease Control and Prevention, National Center for Chronic Disease Prevention and Health Promotion, Atlanta, Ga.

CHAPTER 8

Bandura, A., Social Foundations of Thought and Action: A Social Cognitive Theory, Prentice-Hall International Inc., Englewood Cliffs, N.J., 1986.

Emery, S., Actualizations: You Don't Have to Rehearse to be Yourself, Irvington Publishers, New York, N.Y., 1980.

Greene, G.W., Rossi, S.R., Rossi, J.S., Velicer, W.F., Fava, J.L., and Prochaska, J.O., "Dietary applications of the Stages of Change Model", Journal of the American Dietetic Association, 6:673-678, 1999.

Marcus, B.H., Banspach, S.W., Lefebvre, R.C., Rossi, J.S., Carleton, R.A., and Abrams, D.B., "Using the Stages of Change model to increase the adoption of physical activity among community participants," American Journal of Health Promotion, 6:424-429, 1992.